OXFORD MEDICAL PUBLICATIONS

Efficient Care in General Practice

Efficient Care in General Practice

or: How to look after even more patients

Oxford General Practice Series 21

G. N. MARSH

General Practitioner, Stockton on Tees, Cleveland

OXFORD   NEW YORK   TOKYO
OXFORD UNIVERSITY PRESS
1991

Oxford University Press, Walton Street, Oxford OX2 6DP

Oxford New York Toronto
Delhi Bombay Calcutta Madras Karachi
Petaling Jaya Singapore Hong Kong Tokyo
Nairobi Dar es Salaam Cape Town
Melbourne Auckland

and associated companies in
Berlin Ibadan

Oxford is a trade mark of Oxford University Press

Published in the United States
by Oxford University Press, New York

A catalogue record for this book is available from the British Library

Library of Congress Cataloging in Publication Data
Marsh, G. N. (Geoffrey Norman)
Efficient care in general practice / G. N. Marsh.
(Oxford general practice series ; 21) (Oxford
medical publications)
Includes bibliographical references.
1. Family medicine—Practice. 2. Medical appointments and
schedules. 3. Physicians—Time management. I. Title. II. Series.
III. Series: Oxford general practice series ; no. 21.
[DNLM: 1. Family Practice—organization & administration.
2. Quality Assurance, Health Care—organization & administration.
W1 OX55 no. 21 / W 89 M364e]
R728.M32 1992   610'.68–dc20   91-23983
ISBN 0–19–261953–5 (pbk.)

Typeset by CentraCet, Cambridge
Printed in Great Britain by
Dotesios Ltd
Trowbridge, Wiltshire

Acknowledgements

I express my sincere thanks to the following people:

Dr Keith Boothby, my GP brother-in-law in Peterborough, for suggesting that I write the book—in 1969!

Jane Arundell, my editorial secretary, for patiently coping with endless revisions and obfuscations.

Margaret Hammond, RCGP Librarian, for brilliant referencing.

My patients for tolerating my 'efficiency' across so many years—and still coming back for more.

My partners and countless team members for loyal yet critical support.

My wife . . . for everything.

Author's Note

Throughout this book, 'the doctor' is referred to as 'he' and 'the patient', for the most part, as 'she'. This does not indicate the author's lack of awareness of female doctors or male patients but merely avoids the awkwardness of stating 'he or she' or 'him or her' repeatedly in the text.

Contents

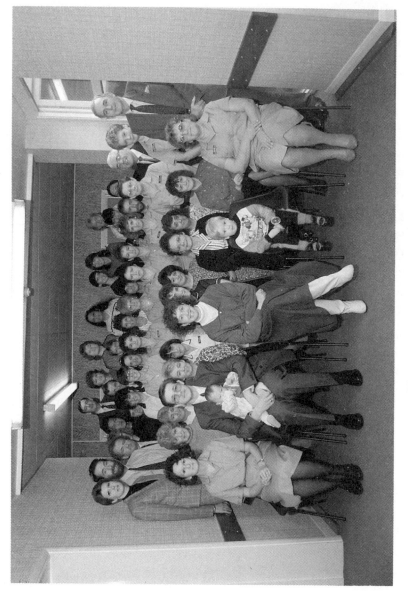

'The primary health-care team, 1991'

Introduction

In 1969 I journeyed to Aberdeen to give the North East Scotland Faculty Lecture of the Royal College of General Practitioners, and I entitled it '5000 Patients—An Easy Life in General Practice'. The audience appeared to be fascinated, the applause was considerable, and from that day to this the average list-size in Aberdeen has fallen from approximately 2500 patients per doctor to about 1500 patients per doctor. So much for the impact of a faculty lecture! It is possible, therefore, that the appeal of this book will be somewhat limited in Aberdeen.

Nevertheless, I have long been interested in the potential for a general practitioner to look after larger rather than smaller numbers of patients, so long as it is done in a caring fashion which is both acceptable to the patients and clinically satisfactory. That is the major theme of this book.

Although the title of the lecture referred to a 5000-list practice, this book should be useful for any size of practice. If its ideas are implemented with a small list, those patients can be cared for in half the time and doctors can take on other jobs as well if they wish—they might even have time to write books. The book will be particularly useful to trainee GPs as yet not set in their ways, and inordinately helpful to overwhelmed principals: the sort of GP who always seems to be late for lunch, doesn't get home early in the evenings, and finds he has visits to do on a half-day. The suggestions in the book will be, of necessity, incomplete. There are very many ways of reducing work-load, and no doubt the reader will have more and better ideas of how to do it than are spelled out here. Nevertheless, by gathering together those I have, I think the book should be a stimulus to thinking about the general concept. Overall, however, I do believe that even the most efficient doctors will find some things that are new or worth a try. And if you really feel I've missed something out, write and tell me—one day there may be a second edition!

At the end of each chapter there are several important references, expertly selected by my colleague Margaret Hammond, Librarian at the Royal College of General Practitioners.

PERSONAL APPROACH

I inherited a list of 3000 patients from an extremely popular and venerated doctor in the early 1960s; I just had to get on and look after them. As I did so, and as I saw alternative ways of continuing to look after all these people, I began to make a virtue of necessity.

At that time, our primary health-care team was beginning to develop. I began to realize the possibility of stretching the potential of individual team members and that this would be the main method of reducing doctor work-load.[1-3] From this followed the whole concept of 'de-doctoring' care. Hence, it will come as no surprise that the first and major chapter in the book is entitled 'Sharing care with other professionals', and that the second chapter is 'Working as a team'.

I have looked at the various components of my day-to-day work and tried to show how I have abbreviated them. Thus the third chapter is on home visits, whose reduction is probably the major method of saving time in general practice. Then as surgery sessions have grown, it has become necessary to refine the work-load on consultations there. This has necessitated chapters on 'efficient' records, the 'efficient' consulting-room, working fast, and using the telephone. In some chapters I lean heavily on the operational research that I have done across the years.

I have always found visits to other practices helpful, and their ways of increasing efficiency, taken for granted there, have often been new to me. I have noted them and adopted them in my own practices. Working with people from other disciplines, particularly those concerned in the management area, has been mind-expanding: for example, I have written papers with accountants, and in conjunction with architects I have designed consulting-rooms and premises.

One of the most important things to realize is that my efficient caring has taken time to effect. The concept of the primary health-care team was boosted by the Family Doctor Charter in the mid 1960s, and now, by the 1990s, the team numbers have trebled and the roles expanded and become more sophisticated.[4,5] But it has taken thirty years, and we are still developing. So for those readers just starting off, remember that it will take time. On the whole, I have found it useful to take one area, or one team member's role, study it, and develop it. Sometimes progress is slow, sometimes in leaps and bounds. Remember also that you cannot expect to implement every point in this book. Some of what I describe does not pertain to our practice—would that it did. Nevertheless, you can try out ideas that appeal to you and hopefully make life a little easier for yourself.

AS A PHILOSOPHY

I was told by a very senior partner shortly after arriving in general practice that good doctors could not be good businessmen. I totally disagree with that, and believe that if one is not a good business person it is difficult to be a good doctor. Caring can be efficient. And yet it is difficult to write a book that concentrates all the time on reducing the doctor's share in caring without seeming to be uncaring. I am not uncaring, and constantly question what I am doing and whether care is improved. I undertook a substantial survey of my own practice in the mid 1970s to discover whether a list of patients seeing their doctor far less frequently than the average—2.3 times per year instead of between 3 and 4 times—would be satisfied with the care given. This forms the second part of my earlier book and was the content of a seminal paper in the *BMJ*.[6] The levels of satisfaction were very high indeed. Put simply, you can be hard-headed without being hard-hearted. And as a final attempt to disarm my critics—you will be sensing my paranoia strongly by now!—at the end of every chapter, I have written a section that examines the efficiency implications of that chapter 'from the patient's point of view'. Sometimes I have merely leaned on my thirty years' experience as a GP, but I have also used the data from my patient-satisfaction survey to substantiate what I have written in the patient's name.

In many walks of life, the importance of productivity and value for money is being stressed. This is also important in medicine, where patients are paying dearly for their care, albeit indirectly and using a free-at-the-time service. However, the provider should not forget that the money is ultimately coming out of the patient's pocket. If people want better roads, expanded social services, and improved schools, to name only three areas, then it is vital that when they are ill their health-care should be cost-effective. In common with many doctors, I have always felt embarrassed about the large number of patients per doctor in Third World countries. How can developed countries like the USA be comfortable with the fact that there are estimated to be about 420 patients per practising doctor,[7] when there are tens of thousands of patients per doctor in poor countries?[8] Indeed, such countries have lessons to teach us since, because of the shortage of doctors, they have learnt to provide care without them.[9]

THE DEBATE

I do not expect any doctor to agree with everything that has been written in this book, or wish to implement all of its ideas; this applies to nurses and other team members too. But I do think that all doctors and team members will find food for thought and, I hope, many useful ideas. Where they do disagree, they should ask themselves whether it is because of custom, conventional wisdom, specific features in their own practice, or plain prejudice and preconditioning. What they decide will indicate what action they could, should, or even will, take.

THE OMISSIONS

For the bulk of the book the emphasis will be on patients' clinical care. Hence, efficient managerial structures for supervising and running the practice, well-ordered accountancy, architects, and lawyers' participation, and so on—although an important background to the book—will not be examined in any detail.

RESULTS OF IMPLEMENTING THESE IDEAS

The final chapter describes the results of having a large list of patients. Paramount is the clinical satisfaction of looking after large numbers of sick people well. To have more time to care more intensively for the more seriously ill must produce clinically contented doctors and also happier co-operating team members. And it must also produce a greater bonding between patient and doctor, as an increasing proportion of serious illness is managed by their known team of carers without the need for referral to hospital and other less-familiar agencies.

FROM THE PATIENT'S POINT OF VIEW

I have shown this Introduction to several patients, a member of my own family, and some of my team colleagues, and the majority of them are prepared to go along with what I have written. As some of my patients have said, people in general equate a well-organized surgery and an efficient and ordered doctor with good care: 'If the "system" is dreadful and disorganized and the doctor is responsible for it then what is his care like?'

Now read on . . .

REFERENCES

1. Marsh, G. N. and Kaim-Caudle, P. (1976). *Team care in general practice.* Croom Helm, London.
2. Marsh, G. N. and McNay, R. A. (1974). Team workload in an English general practice. *British Medical Journal*, **1**, 315–18.
3. Marsh, G. N. and McNay, R. A. (1974). Factors affecting workload in general practice. *British Medical Journal*, **1**, 319–22.
4. British Medical Association (1965). *Charter for the family doctor.* BMA, London.
5. Department of Health (1990). Statistics for general medical practitioners in England and Wales: 1978 to 1988. *Statistical Bulletin*, **4**, 9, 15.
6. Kaim-Caudle, P. R. and Marsh, G. N. (1975). Patient satisfaction survey in general practice. *British Medical Journal*, **1**, 262–4.
7. Hiatt, H. H. (1987). *America's health in the balance. Choice or chance?* Harper and Row, New York.

8. Joseph, A. E. and Phillips, D. R. (1984). *Accessibility and Utilization, Geographical perspectives in health care delivery*. Harper and Row, New York.
9. Morley, D., Rohde, J. E., and Williams, G. (ed.). *Practising health for all*. Oxford University Press.

1. Sharing care with fellow professionals

THE PRIMARY HEALTH-CARE TEAM

As I stated in the Introduction, the sharing of care within the team has been, and still is, one of the major ways that doctors have cared more efficiently for their patients with less personal effort from themselves. Hence the primacy of this chapter. The possibility of developing teams of doctors, nurses, health-visitors, and so on, was considered as far back as the 1920s when the building of health centres was first proposed.[1] But it was only from the mid-1960s that doctors really began to come together in groups in either their own practice premises or local authority health centres. The concept of what came to be known as the primary health-care team was boosted by two major steps: the reimbursement of 70 per cent of the wages of their employed staff to the doctors, and the attachment to the practices of all the nursing staff that had previously worked for local authorities under the jurisdiction of the medical officers of health.[2] Early photographs taken between the mid-1960s and the mid 1970s of the primary health-care team showed the doctors seated in the front row and the supporting staff gathered behind them like rays from the sun. To my own chagrin I had toured the USA in 1974 as a visiting professor proclaiming the virtues of this British team phenomenon.[3] I was told firmly yet diplomatically that it looked to the Americans, and particularly to non-doctor female Americans, like a nasty, male-chauvinist, professional, hierarchical piggery! In fact they were largely right.

Opposite page 1 of the Introduction to this book, you will see a primary health-care team of the 1990s. Central to it are the patients, who take an appropriate place in the front row, and behind them are scattered a democratic mix of caring fellow professionals, each with a high regard for the training and expertise of the other. Because of the praiseworthy increase in the number of female doctors into general practice, coinciding with their almost 50 per cent output from British medical schools, the team includes female doctors. Although in functional terms, as well as in photographic ones, the doctors may have lost much of their pivotal role, it must be emphasized that by virtue of their contracts doctors must provide ample open access to their consulting sessions for all their patients. Thus the patient need never be daunted by this panoply of carers, but will know that an appointment-system with her doctor available is always hers to use. Frequently the doctor works as a signpost to the team, filtering off those patients for whom only he can care, and directing to others in the team inappropriate problems or problems for which team members have greater expertise than the doctor. Indeed, fundamental to team care must be the early and ready acceptance by the doctor that he does not know everything, and that others in the team know better. The doctor is taught to diagnose in physical, psychological, and social terms, but it is probable that a very large proportion of the patients with psychological and social components to their problems can receive better care from others in the team. Purely physical problems will need his clinical expertise, but even then many of the investigations and much of the routine, ongoing care of physical illness can be shared with the various types of nurse within the team. Chapter 7 will emphasize that preventative care is largely the task of the nursing members of the team.

The doctor's provision of continual access to all patients does not preclude patients seeking direct access to other members of the team whom they may feel more appropriate to their problem (for example, a child's feeding problem which might be best treated by a health-visitor). Indeed, the enlightened-practice brochure may well have more detailed descriptions of non-doctor care within its pages, and how to seek it out, than detail about the provision of medical care (see Chapter 14).[4] Patients must be given choice as to whom they consult. Having once received care from non-doctors in the team, it frequently transpires that where that care has been effective, patients will return to them for similar problems.

Three major points emerge: first, that the doctor remembers his team colleagues when he is consulting, and shares patients' care accordingly; secondly, that the patients are educated by brochures, newsletters, trained (or at least informed) receptionists, and so on, as to who the team are and when they are available; and thirdly, that the team members themselves make themselves suitably accessible. How the team actually works together is the subject of Chapter 2. It must be remembered that the fellow professional colleagues of the doctors are highly trained, and look forward to using their knowledge to the full and even having their role extended.

So who are all these people in the team-photograph? They can be divided into seven major groups.

1. Reception, records, and computer staff

Filing clerks	Receptionists
Computer clerks	Records analyst
Computer and records supervisor	

Among the responsibilities of the above group is that of ensuring a steady flow of patients to the doctor and other members of the team when they are consulting. The contents of the record should be efficiently date-ordered, something which can be achieved with difficulty in the FP5 and 6 record envelope, and more easily in A4 folders.[5–8] Increasingly the patient's record will be on computer and visually displayed on each doctor's desk (see Chapter 10). Whatever the system, missing records, the wrong record, inaccurate data, and faulty or slow computers all militate against efficiency. Increasingly the doctor or nurse will be able to display on a desk-top computer summary sheets of major illnesses, preventative-care procedures, day-to-day clinical notes, and laboratory investigations, to all of which he will add by tapping appropriate keys, or have someone available after his surgery to do it for him. Only when he needs all this data away from his consulting room—for example, when doing home visits—will he need a printout to take with him.

The efficiency and expertise of receptionists at the 'shop-window' of the practice is vital.[9,10] They have a major role in facilitating the patient's access to doctors and other team members, and informing these team members when 'bottlenecks' or waiting-lists are developing. They have an important role in educating patients as to whom they should see, and this will be reinforced in the practice brochure. They can be a major help to the doctor in relaying messages from him to patients. Essential to this role is a thorough understanding of the practice and how it functions. Although many receptionists now attend courses about their job, or are trained at colleges of education prior to starting, it is essential that they meet together, under the tutelage of the practice manager, to discuss the philosophies and day-to-day working of their own particular practice.[11–13] My own practice now closes every Thursday for two hours at lunchtime for this staff-training. Efficiency must begin at the practice 'shop-window'.

2. Office and administration staff

Cleaners	Tea-lady
Switchboard operator	Office juniors
Secretaries	Practice manager

The tasks of the members of the above group will be apparent from their title, but one of the most important of them is the tea-lady, who should aim to provide a better cup of tea or coffee within the premises than is available anywhere else in the surrounding town. This will improve the ambience at team meetings and facilitate communications.

The role of the practice manager has increased enormously in recent years, and her job description is too complicated to spell out here; there is now a considerable literature about it.[14–16] By co-ordinating the whole operation of the team, and also by working with accountants, architects, solicitors, and the more senior members of the Family Health Services

Authority (formerly FPC), she can relieve the doctors of much of the work that they did previously. The creation of a new appointments system, computerization of the day-to-day salaries and accounts, evaluation of the need for adding a new wing to the premises, and financial implications for the practice of a senior partner undertaking twenty-four-hour retirement, not to mention the many many machinations of the implications of the 'new contract' and the White Paper, including the implementation and monitoring of fund-holding, are all under her jurisdiction. She has an important role in pouring oil on the troubled waters of any interpersonal conflicts within the team; this does not exclude the doctors. Her training and expertise must be of the highest, and her salary will be appropriate. A recent practice-manager vacancy for a group practice in the North of England was advertised at £23 000 per annum. Some practice managers are becoming shareholding partners.

The switchboard operator should be the efficient signpost to the team, and not merely a receptionist answering the phone as best she can. Her tone of voice should be welcoming and calmly professional. Her aim should be an immediate answer to all callers, even if she has to put some on 'hold' while earlier callers are dealt with. The aura of efficiency created by an immediate response on the telephone is eminently worth encouraging.

The overall aim of the managerial and secretarial 'office' group is that, by working efficiently and in a co-ordinated way, they can relieve the other team members, and particularly the doctors, of a large number of tasks and a massive amount of 'hassle'.

3. The nursing team

Community-nursing sisters*   Community midwife*
Community enrolled nurses*   Health-visitors*
Practice nurses   School nurse*
Family-Planning nurse   MacMillan nurse
Community psychiatric nurse*
Psychogeriatric nurse*
Drug-and-alcohol abuse counsellor*
(* District Health Authority employees attached to practices)

The nurses are the powerhouse of the team. In terms of total work-load, it is probable that their combined output exceeds that of the doctors. By carrying out their own nursing roles effectively, and expanding and increasing their potential as doctors increasingly use their skills, they become fundamental to producing efficient care in general practice. Under each nurse's heading in the next few pages is a list of her tasks, orientating more particularly on areas where they can reduce the doctors' work-load.

Community-nursing sister

Community nurses are mature, highly trained nurses with expertise equivalent to senior ward sisters in hospital. A significant proportion of their time is spent on home visits, particularly to the elderly, house-bound, and chronically sick. Their day-to-day practical nursing should largely be delegated to the attached state-enrolled community nurses—for example, dressings, some injections, general nursing care, etc.. Thus they can share a great deal of the consultative visiting of the chronic house-bound elderly sick with the doctor (see Chapter 3). Their work in the practice premises alongside the community state-enrolled nurses includes a therapeutic area—for example, dressings, injections, ear syringe, and so on—a diagnostic area—for example, venepunctures, throat swabs, ECGs etc., and unusually (for many of them do not have the time), the running of diabetic, vascular, geriatric, and preventative-care clinics.[17] There is no doubt that the volume and quality of work undertaken in the premises by the attached community nurses has an enormous effect on the remaining work to be done by the practice nurse. Patently, the more that the attached nurses can do the less there is for the practice nurse to do. Currently there is a great variation in the work done by community nurses from one practice to another and from one district or region to another.

Practice nurse

Table 1.1 gives some indication of the type of care being undertaken by an experienced practice nurse in our 15 000 patient practice. She sees approximately 500 patients per month, many of whom were previously seen by doctors before she became a member of the team in the late 1960s.[18,19] She sees about 100 patients for each doctor each month. The highest percentage of the work is preventative (68 per cent), followed by therapeutic at 24 per cent. The volume of work under the various detailed headings in Table 1.1 has varied across the years. The trend has been for 'clinic-style' work to start slowly as appropriate patients were detected and referred by their doctors. Yet even after two or three years, a significant number of diabetics were not attending the clinic regularly. It is essential that all team members remember that the clinics exist and, when opportunities present, direct patients to them. In both preventative and therapautic areas the nurse works to protocols which have been designed by nurse herself in consultation with the other nurses in the practice and her doctor colleagues. The therapeutic and preventative-care protocols are discussed later (Chapters 4 and 7). Even at this level of care she is not functioning as a nurse-practitioner since, apart from the odd occasion, she does not work as a diagnostician. My definition of a nurse-practitioner is a nurse who does all the above work, plus some antenatal care and child development (areas covered in Britain by the midwife and health-visitor), and in

Table 1.1   *Practice-nurse audit, 1989*

Procedure or clinic	Number of patients	% of patients per procedure	% of patients per group
Preventative work			68
Well-woman clinic	554	9	
Cervical smears	1046	18	
Well-man clinic	301	5	
Tetanus and travel injections	1199	21	
Immunizations	890	15	
Diagnostic			8
Venipunctures and swabs	445	8	
Therapeutic work			24
Medical 'extras'	220	4	
Surgical 'extras'	180	3	
Miscellaneous injections	338	6	
Clinics			
Diabetic	276	5	
Vascular	117	2	
Minor ops	251	4	
TOTAL	5817	100	100

addition sees unfiltered medical problems necessitating diagnostic skills.[20,21] Usually she has had specific training in history-taking of the undifferentiated problem, as well as in physical examination using torch, auriscope, stethoscope, tendon hammer, and so on. This diagnostic work differentiates the nurse-practitioner from the practice nurse. There have been experiments with nurse-practitioners in Great Britain, and they were fairly commonplace in the USA and Canada in the 1970s. Enthusiasm for them has waned in America, and the tradition in this country of seeing a doctor 'to find out what's the matter' dies hard.[22,23] In my own practice there have been so many other areas for the practice nurse to fill that the effort of developing her diagnostic role has remained at the bottom of the agenda. There is no doubt, however, that a 'minor illness' nurse advising on home care of minor problems—coughs, colds, sore throats, diarrhoea, aches and pains and the like, could indeed reduce the doctors' work-load considerably.[24] With the need for larger lists of patients per doctor, this could be one area ripe for experimentation and development in the 1990s.

Community midwife
The attached community midwife, frequently working with pupil midwives and supported by a practice receptionist, can run the antenatal and

postnatal clinics for the practice.[25] She is fully able to undertake the continuing care of normal women. She needs a doctor available principally to deal with diagnostic problems, variations from the norm, prescribing of therapy, and as 'psychological' support from time to time during the pregnancy. Antenatal care is essentially preventative, and the reduced programme and individually styled care is described later (Chapter 7).

Family-planning nurse

Women wishing to start contraception, and those already using it, can be assessed and advised by trained family-planning nurses, employed by practices.[18] Alternatively, the work can be undertaken by appropriately trained community-nursing sisters or community midwives, but time is their main constraint.

Health-visitors

Traditionally the health-visitor has been the mainstay of preventative care in the community (see Chapter 7). Perhaps because general practitioners have not appreciated the important role of health-visitors and the valuable work they can take off their shoulders, suitable accommodation has not always been made available for them, particularly in privately owned group practices.[26] Health-visitors need rooms of their own in which to keep their records, organize their work, and consult their clients. They also need large rooms for their preventative work with groups, and for child-health clinics. As for all other members of the team, suitable accommodation makes for more efficient working and greater job satisfaction.

School nurse

In areas where a practice team's paediatric patients all attend one or two schools in the district, it seems sensible for the school nurse to liaise regularly with that team. In my own practice, the experiment of having the school nurse based in the practice and doing her clinics at the nearby schools, thus facilitating liaison with the GPs and health-visitors, have proved reasonably successful. Such experiments are worth repeating.

MacMillan nurse

These nurses concern themselves with the dying and their families.[27] Initially, when they began to liaise with our team we felt affronted. Care of the dying had always been done, or so we thought, with commitment and dedication, including frequent home visits by doctor or nurses. What more could the specialist nurses offer? In effect what they offered was greater expertise in the therapeutic management of the difficult symptoms of dying people, like anergy, nausea, bone pain, repetitive vomiting, and so on. If they themselves did not have suggestions to make to our team, they contacted their 'experts'—often people working at hospices (initially in London, but now our local hospice)—and got further advice. In addition, they are aware of all supporting services that can be provided in a particular community, and they mobilize them. In no way have they made any members of our team feel redundant but have complemented the services already being offered. As a result of their presence, more people now die more comfortably in their own homes, and their carers are the more fulfilled.

Community psychiatric nurse

Increasingly these nurses have been attached to group practices.[28,29] In addition to their traditional continuing, chronic care of the psychotics in the practice—schizophrenics, agoraphobes, chronic recurrent depressives, and so on—they also provide valuable ongoing supervisory care of patients with acute psychiatric illnesses. A patient with newly diagnosed depression or anxiety-state or obsessive neurosis can be visited at home a day or two after the initial doctor consultation. Their psychotropic drugs can be monitored, and modified if necessary, and in addition the nurse can provide insight, education, guidance and counselling, as well as reporting the patient's progress to the doctor. The visiting of patients who have taken overdoses and patients discharged from in-patient care is another part of their work. By remembering to share care with the community psychiatric-nursing staff, many of whom have held posts as senior charge nurses and sisters in psychiatric units, as well as having received community-based education and experience, the general practitioner can provide more comprehensive and detailed care for his psychiatric patients without extra effort himself. As the community psychiatric nurse's work-load increases, she requires consulting-room facilities at the surgery.

Psychogeriatric nurse

The psychogeriatric nurse has a similar role to the community psychiatric nurse except that she deals with patients over the age of 65. Accordingly, a large and important volume of her work concerns itself with dementia. By marrying together the doctor's clinical assessment and the psychogeriatric nurse's functional assessment (Hodkinson memory-information tests, and so on), a comprehensive picture can be drawn of the degree of dementia and appropriate therapy and management instituted. The care facilities available in the district (day hospitals, luncheon clubs, 'outings', carers support groups, and so on), will be well known to the community psychogeriatric nurse and can be utilized. The often prolonged care, the monitoring of deterioration, and ultimate admission to appropriate residential home of demented patients was formerly an onerous task for the general practitioner. Much of this is now done by the psychogeriatric nurse. Although a large proportion of the nurse's work concerns itself with dementia, she also provides care and supervision of other older psychiatric patients in the practice—paraphrenics, depressives, obsessives, and so on—frequently employing counselling and relaxation techniques. Indeed, it is important that the proportion of her work with dements does not become too great, and that it is interspersed with other psychoses of the elderly, especially those of a remediable nature, otherwise the job would become untenable.

Drug-and-alcohol abuse counsellor

The explosion of psychotropic-drug therapy in the 1960s and 1970s has left a residue of addicted patients. By careful analysis of computerized or even manual records—or just from memory or repeat prescriptions—these patients can be identified. By giving the drug-and-alcohol abuse counsellor access to a consulting-room, she can supervise their continuing care with the ultimate aim of stopping their drugs. There are many reasons why alcoholics, or just 'heavy drinkers', are not identified by their general practitioners, but one is the feeling of helplessness that many GPs have as to what to do about them once they are diagnosed. For the GP to have a member of the team available to treat (counsel) these patients, either individually or in groups, makes their detection much more meaningful. The doctor's role is identification (diagnosis) and clinical assessment, but the ongoing care can be shared, and often largely taken over, by a trained drug-and-alcohol abuse counsellor.

4. Advisers: non-medical and non-nursing

Social worker   Dietitian
Physiotherapist   Counsellor
Elderly-care visitor   Patients' association secretary
Breast-feeding counsellor

The above group are all trained professionals, albeit customarily without nursing or medical qualifications.

Social worker

Analyses of the content of GP consultations across the years and in many studies have shown that there is an enormous influx of social problems to general practitioners.[30,31] Most frequently they envelop and aggravate the clinical problems, but sometimes patients will consult their doctors on purely social matters. This applies particularly to the socially deprived. Uncommonly, practices have a social worker attached entirely to them, but most have an informal liaison with a social-work team, and not unusually the same person attends the practice and consults by appointment. Amongst the common problems are housing, finance, isolation (loneliness), grants, home-helps, social requests for abortion, and aids for the disabled. There is no doubt that the resolution of social problems reduces the doctor's work, but, like chronic medical conditions, social problems are often not 'curable'. However, concern and care about them certainly reduces the ensuing morbidity.

Dietitian

Regular weekly attendance by a dietitian relieves the doctor of much of the continuing care of patients with diet-related conditions.[32,33] Increasingly, her expertise is being used for:

(a) diabetics

(b) other illnesses requiring special dietary advice: for example, malabsorption, anorexia, irritable bowel syndrome, and so on;

(c) patients with organic disease which is being seriously worsened by weight problems, such as arthritis, ischaemic heart disease, and so on;

(d) the obese.

The conditions are listed in this order because there is no doubt that dietitians would be overwhelmed and find little job satisfaction if all overweight patients were referred to them. For the most part, the overweight patient does not require the expertise of a dietitian but merely some sensible advice from doctor or nurse, appropriate diet-and-exercise programmes, and encouragement to attend weight-watcher groups in the area. This, perhaps dismissive, view of the obese comes from increasing disillusionment over many years with my lack of success at reducing my patients' weight and keeping it reduced.

Physiotherapist

Only rarely do practices have physiotherapy facilities.[34,35] In the main, these are provided at the local hospital via a long waiting-list to see a consultant. Because of this delay, most physiotherapy is given to chronic conditions. As one of a group of fund-holding practices, we liaised with the senior physiotherapist at the local hospital with regard to paying her some of our development grant. For this amount, she has arranged for a physiotherapy session at each of the practices at a specified time each week. Access to them is either direct or via the GP. Certainly much of the medicating of acute physical illness can be replaced by physiotherapeutic measures, frequently with greater and speedier benefit and with no risk of iatrogenic disease.

Elderly-care visitor

Although the community nurses are involved with the care of the elderly on a day-to-day nursing basis, as well as in a consultative way, there is no doubt that the trained elderly-care visitor, aware of the patient's clinical problems and working to a largely social protocol, is of tremendous preventative value (see Chapter 7).[36-38] Family Health Service Authorities have accepted that her annual assessment of the over seventy-fives satisfies the regulations of the 'new contract'.

Counsellor

At least 10 per cent of practices now have a counsellor working on a consultative basis. Many of them have been trained in marriage guidance (now Relate), and have expanded their work from that background.[39] Some have special expertise in psycho-sexual problems. There is no doubt that many of the long, difficult, and emotionally charged consultations that GPs used to have with their unhappy, disaffected (particularly married female) patients can now be much more expertly undertaken by trained counsellors.[40] Again, facilities—a consulting-room with appropriate ambience—must be provided, together with sensitized receptionists to make appointments and receive the patients. When a counsellor first starts in a practice, it is probably necessary for her to indicate the types of problems she perceives as being appropriate for her skills. Marital or partner disharmony will be self-evident, but most types of interpersonal conflict (parent/child, employer/employee, and son on) can benefit from counselling. Loss of self-esteem and other problems with self-image constitute the largest group of conditions in my own practice. Although the number of clients that a counsellor may see in any group practice is often relatively small, the chronicity of their problems and the length of time taken to counsel them often saves the doctor hours of consultations. Furthermore, the expertise of trained counsellors far exceeds anything that the great majority of general practitioners can offer. This is one member of the team from whom patients will seek further appointments directly, without consulting their general practitioner again.

5. The doctors

In order to complete the identification of all the people in the team-photograph, is is necessary to say that there are seven list-holding principals—six full-time, one part-time—as well as two trainees.

6. Occasional members

Community medical officers (child-health)   Architects
Ministers of religion   Solicitor
Accountants

Community medical officers

The overlap in the care of children, and particularly for the deprived and the handicapped, between community medical officers (child-health) and general practitioners is considerable. Integration and the avoidance of duplication of care can be facilitated if the CMO occasionally attends team meetings. In some practices, community medical officers have become part of the extended primary health-care team, taking responsibility for immunization programmes, developmental paediatrics, and the like.

Ministers of religion

Churchmen have cared for the sick across the centuries—for much longer than doctors—and their expert counselling skills are welcome in the care of the dying, the bereaved, and the suddenly seriously ill. Familiarity with the faces and 'styles' of the various ministers of different denominations aids communication, and their occasional presence at the informal morning-coffee meeting facilitates this (see Chapter 2).

Accountant, architect, and solicitor

Financial viability of the team is crucial, so a good, involved accountant is obviously vital. He becomes even more important in fund-holding practices and works closely with the practice manager. The architect occasionally, and the solicitor hopefully very little (except perhaps for updating the practice agreement) are fellow professionals needed from time to time.

7. Missing people

Pharmacist   Chiropodist
Dentist   Optician
Acupuncturist   Hypnotist

Pharmacist

There are very few reported experiments of pharmacists working closely with primary health-care teams.[41,42] Our own sudden decision to cease prescribing for minor illness caused considerable problems for the pharmacists in the area.[43] They had large stocks of previously prescribed preparations and suddenly no market. Closer liaison and joint planning could have avoided the problem.

One method of reducing the volume of minor illness that presents itself to general practitioners would be to increase the role of the pharmacists. One duty Sunday morning I visited my local chemist to obtain some urgent drugs and overheard the requests of patients for medication either for themselves or their relatives. The 'histories' were recounted to relatively junior chemists' assistants, and were almost identical to many that I listen to in the consulting-room. The response was the selling of preparations for symptom relief. Thus minor illness was dealt with on a Sunday. It seemed to me that if this system was encouraged and welcomed by doctor and pharmacist respectively, then patients would increasingly use it. It will come as no surprise that our practice brochure positively recommends patients to consult our nearest pharmacist about minor problems. The pharmacist of the future could be the person who will ultimately shoulder much of the burden of minor illness that currently consults general practitioners.

Chiropodist

Chiropodists sometimes work in health centres but very rarely in privately owned group-practice centres. However, as the latter become fund-holding, there will be opportunities to involve chiropodists in the day-to-day care of patients. Verrucas, ingrowing toenails, bunions, plantar fasciitis, flat feet, crossed toes, and so on, currently common problems for GPs, could all be directed to chiropodists if they were available.

Dentist

It seems odd that dental care and medical care have been so widely separated, and their closer liaison could well be beneficial. Time for experiment?

Optician

As the management of diabetes and hypertension increasingly becomes a general practitioner task, the need for an expert opinion of the condition of the retina becomes more vital. Squint—or query squint—in children, is a not uncommon GP problem. A good working relationship with a local optician, including the provision of eye reports on individual patients, could improve care without extra effort or expertise from the general practitioner himself, and also obviate the need for secondary referral to hospital eye departments. Experiments along these lines are occurring in some group practices, and need analysis and recording.

Acupuncturists, hypnotists, and the like

Again, fund-holding practices may wish to experiment with care by these people. Their training, expertise, and the protocols to which they work would have to be scrutinized by the doctors since problems of responsibility might arise. Another area for interesting experiments.

SHARING CARE WITH FELLOW PROFESSIONALS FROM THE PATIENT'S POINT OF VIEW

There is no doubt that, so long as patients know they can have prompt access to their own doctor, they appreciate the other services that can be provided alongside him. Above all they welcome the additional expertise. In my own patient-satisfaction survey, although a high degree of satisfaction with the doctor was evinced, there was an even higher degree of satisfaction with the nursing care; this applied to midwife and health-visitor also.

Patients appreciate good communication between doctors, nurses, mid-wives, and others and certainly sense when this is not taking place. Occasional joint visits by doctor and community nurse to the chronic house-bound sick are particularly well received. Patients welcome the oppportunities provided by multiple types of carer, and are relieved that they do not always have to 'bother the doctor'. Sharing care with fellow professionals should mean better and more comprehensive treatment.

REFERENCES

1. Davison Report (1920). *Interim report on the future provision of medical and allied services*. HMSO, London.
2. British Medical Association (1965). *Charter for the family doctor*. BMA, London.
3. Marsh, G. N. (1975). Primary Medical Care—The co-operative solution to the volume problem. *Journal of the American Medical Association*.
4. Marsh, G. N. (1980). The practice brochure: a patient's guide to team care. *British Medical Journal*, **281**, 730–2.
5. Zander, L. I., Beresford, S. A. A. and Thomas, P. (1978). *Medical records in general practice*. Occasional paper No. 5. RCGP London.
6. Marsh, G. N. and Thornham, J. R. (1980). Changing to A4 folders and updating records in a 'busy' general practice. *British Medical Journal*, **281**, 215–17.
7. Acheson, H. W. K. (1976). Converting medical records to A4 size in general practice. *Journal of the Royal College of General Practitioners*, **26**, 277–81
8. Department of Health and Social Security (1974). *Joint working party on re-design of medical records in general practice*. Interim report. HMSO, London.
9. Drury, M. and Collin, M. (1986). *The medical secretary's and receptionist's handbook*, 5th ed. Bailliere, London.
10. Hallsworth, D. (1988). *A handbook for medical receptionists*. Parthenon, Cornforth.
11. Drury, M. (1988). *The practice receptionists' programme*. Radcliffe, Oxford.
12. Whalen, M. (ed.) (1989). *The practice receptionist's programme*, Book 2. Radcliffe, Oxford.
13. Sharp, A. J. H. *et al.* (1989). An assessment of the value of video recordings

of receptionists. *Journal of the Royal College of General Practitioners*, **39**, 421–2.

14. Drury, M. (ed.) (1990). *The new practice manager*. Radcliffe, Oxford.
15. Nelson, E. G. (1976). The role of practice manager—changes in attitudes promoted by the Royal College of General Practitioners. *Journal of the Royal College of General Practitioners*, **26**, 281–91.
16. Pritchard, P., Low, K., and Whalen, M. (1984). *Management in general practice*. Oxford University Press.
17. Dunnell, K. and Dobbs, J. (1982). *Nurses working in the community*. HMSO, London.
18. Marsh, G. N. (1976) Further nursing care in general practice. *British Medical Journal*, **2**, 626–7.
19. Garvie, D. (1990). Sharing Care with a practice nurse. *Horizons* (Oct. 1990).
20. Spitzer, W. D. *et al.* (1974). The Burlington randomized trial of the nurse practitioner. *New England Journal of Medicine*, **290**, 251–6.
21. Bowling, A. and Stilwell, B. (eds) (1988). *The nurse in family practice. Practice nurses and nurse practitioners in primary health care*. Saitari Press, London.
22. Stilwell, B., Greenfield, S., Drury, M., and Hull, F. M. (1987). A nurse practitioner in general practice: working style and pattern of consultations. *Journal of the Royal College of General Practitioners*, **37**, 154–7.
23. Drury, M. Greenfield, S., Stillwell, B., and Hull, F. M. (1988). A nurse practitioner in general practice: patient perceptions and expectations. *Journal of the Royal College of General Practitioners*, **38**, 503–5.
24. Marriott, R. G. (1981). Open access to the practice nurse. *Journal of the Royal College of General Practitioners*, **31**, 235–8.
25. Marsh, G. N. (ed.) (1985). *Modern obstetrics in general practice*. Oxford University Press.
26. Marsh, G. N., Russell, D., and Russell, I. T. (1989). What do health visitors contribute to the care of children? A study in the north of England. *Journal of the Royal College of General Practitioners*, **39**, 201–5.
27. Spilling, R. (ed.) (1986). *Terminal care at home*. Oxford University Press.
28. Marks, I. (1985). Controlled trial of psychiatric nurse therapists in primary care. *British Medical Journal*, **290**, 1181–4.
29. Robertson, H. and Sutt, D. J. (1985). Community psychiatric nursing: a survey of patients and problems. *Journal of the Royal College of General Practitioners*, **35**, 130–2.
30. Huntington, J. (1981). *Social work and general medical practice. Collaboration or conflict?* Allen and Unwin, London.
31. Corney, R. H. (1985). Social work in general practice. *Journal of the Royal College of General Practitioners*, **35**, 291–2.
32. Massey-Lynch, M. (1975). Dietitian in the practice. *Practice Team*, **47**, 8–10.
33. Creager, R. J. Turner, J. M., and Cook, J. E. (1984). The clincial dietitian in family practice residency programs. *Journal of Family Practice*, **18**, 320–4.
34. Pogson, J. and Wilson, J. B. (1981). Physiotherapy in a rural practice. *Practitioner*, **226**, 557–8.
35. Hackett, G. I. Hudson, M. F., Wylie, J. B. *et al*, (1987). Evaluation of the efficacy and acceptability to patients of a physiotherapist working in a health centre. *British Medical Journal*, **294**, 24–6.
36. McIntosh, I. B., Young, M., and Steward, T. (1988). General practice geriatric surveillance scheme. *Scottish Medical Journal*, **33**, 332–3.

37. McIntosh, I. (1990). Primary care specialists or lay visitors for the over-75s screening? *Geriatric Medicine*, **20(4)**, 14, 17.
38. McLeod, J. (1987). *Preventive care of the elderly*, Occasional Paper No. 35. RCGP, London.
39. Marsh, G. N. and Barr, J. (1975). Marriage guidance counselling in a group practice. *Journal of the Royal College of General Practitioners*, **25**, 73–5.
40. McLeod, J. (1988). *The work of counsellors in general practice*. Occasional Paper No. 37. RCGP, London.
41. Shulman, J. I., Shulman, S., and Haines, A. P. (1981). The prevention of adverse drug reactions—a potential role for pharmacists in the primary care team? *Journal of the Royal College of General Practitioners*, **31**, 429–34.
42. Marsland, D. (1987). *Pharmacists and doctors, a study of dispensing in the countryside*. Brunel Institute of Organisation and Social Studies, Uxbridge.
43. Marsh, G. N. (1977). 'Curing' minor illness in general practice. *British Medical Journal*, **2**, 1267–9.

2.   Working as a team

Before considering exactly how that enormous panoply of carers shown in the team-photograph manages to work as a team, it is perhaps necessary to examine briefly its major functions. The primary one must be to work as a 'service' team. It is there to provide care for the innumerable problems that a community brings to its local health centre or group practice. The membership of the team should reflect as closely as possible the demography of the population that it serves; hence, a community with large numbers of mothers with small children should have proportionately more health-visitors. Put simply, the main function of any team should be to look after the people that come to it. Secondly, the team should have a teaching function. Mutual education of fellow professionals on each other's role is automatic when they work alongside each other and communications are good. Each type of carer will have students: doctors will have trainee GPs and medical students, nurses will have students, midwives will have pupils, and health-visitors will have trainee health-visitors. Particularly in areas of high unemployment, receptionists, secretaries, and computer staff will have trainees from various youth (and mature) employment-training schemes. Thirdly, the team can have an audit-and-research function, and in that area the records clerks, records analyst, and computer staff will have major roles.

FACILITIES AND MINI-CLINICS

It will be self-evident that appropriate accommodation is essential for the provision of team care. Many of the workers, for example, counsellors, require only a consulting-room, but others, such as health-visitors and midwives, require more clinic-style facilities. Nevertheless, appropriate expansion of premises brings its own reward by increasing the volume of work that people can do, and could be a worthwhile investment. Between 1966 and 1990, 30 per cent improvement grants were available towards new buildings as well as rent for expanded premises. Under the terms of the 1990 NHS changes, expansion of practice premises will be financed by a development fund. A pump-priming £15 million was allocated initially— a niggardly amount. It is almost certain that much of the future expansion of practice premises and facilities will have to flow from economies in the practice budget. Efficient prescribing will be one particular area in which savings can be made.

RECORDS

A comprehensive, date-ordered, 'communal' record, either manual or on desk-top computer screens, to which each team member can contribute can be of great benefit in co-ordinating individual efforts and encouraging a team spirit. The DHSS A4 folder is excellent for team care, containing as it does separate records for day-to-day clinical notes, nurse and health-visitor notes, records of contraception, antenatal sheets, and sheets for preventative health procedures.[1] Missing data can be identified by lay staff working to a protocol and highlighted on the front of the folder, or the VDU screen, for appropriate members of the team to note and rectifiy whenever the patient presents. By reading the contributions of other team members, communication from one to another is improved. Increasingly, the patients themselves must be aware of what is written in their records or entered on the computer, and be allowed to ordain what is recorded and, perhaps more importantly, what is not.

JOINT CARING

Detailed and important communication takes place where two members of the team work together on the same problem. For example, doctor and midwife get to know and understand each other's working-methods well when caring for patients in labour, and perhaps more frequently when working in the same premises at a shared antenatal clinic. Similarly, the doctor and community nurses who meet by pre-arrangement at the patient's home to inspect dressings or look at wounds develop close working links. Doctor and health-visitor frequently work side by side at developmental paediatric clinics (see Chapter 7). This day-to-day sharing of clinical areas bonds members of the team together, co-ordinates their work, and minimizes duplication.

The more that patients perceive practices working as a team the more they will come to equate care by one team member with care by them all.[2] 'I know the nurse will inform the doctor if things aren't going right or I need more treatment'—a quote from my patient-satisfaction survey.[3] Occasional joint visits inculcate this feeling and in fact reduce duplicated care, always something to be aware of when working in a team.

MEETINGS

Ideally, each member of the team should know how to reach any other member virtually at any time. The receptionists' knowledge here is vital and it is they who will know more than anyone how people can be contacted. From moment to moment, it is the receptionists who will be called upon to arrange contact. Continuously throughout the day, in the rooms and corridors of the premises, there will be constant communication between team members 'bumping into each other'. Nevertheless, there do need to be formal opportunities for communications, and hence a plethora of meetings of various types. Time spent at them must be as brief as possible—the 'work' still remains to be done!

The morning meeting

Each morning the team will meet together, preferably sitting around a table in a degree of comfort and with coffee and tea available. Liaising members of large teams like the one in the team-photograph, will obviously not all meet every day, but an 'inner core' of doctors, nurses, health-visitors, midwife, and practice manager should try to meet almost daily. Counsellors, dietitians, social workers, and so on have regular days when they are known to attend, and relevant problems can be kept until then. Central to the meeting will be the requests for home visits that will have been assembled by the receptionists early in the morning for the various team members. Some common-rooms now have three or four telephones within them because of patients' demand for telephone advice (see Chapter 13). Thus there will be a general hubbub arising from telephone conversations as well as discussions between team members utilizing the notes of the patient with the problem. It should be noted incidentally that cross-referral of problems does not need to involve doctors at all: midwives liaise frequently with health-visitors and they in turn with counsellors and social workers. Above all, this meeting needs to be short, no longer than twenty minutes, completely informal, and very much concerned with the day-to-day problems of individual patients.

House committee meeting

The house committee consists of the doctors, practice and community nurses, midwife, health-visitors, practice manager, records and computer systems supervisor, and the senior receptionist. The meetings, which can be held approximately once a month (perhaps over an 'interesting lunch'— if the practice budget permits), serve to weld the team into a functioning unit. Topics discussed are for the most part operational and clinical, and health-visitors, midwives, nurses, and doctors talking together can formulate policies on various aspects of care. Subjects as varied as breast-feeding, room availability, cigarette smoking, appointment times, alcoholics, immunization rates, 'targets', minor-ops clinics, training programmes, welcoming of new members, patients' groups meetings, attitude to minor illness, and so on, have all been discussed at our house committee within the last two years. It is as a result of these meetings that the general aims of the team can be developed and its overall philosophy can emerge. At these meetings individual members from various disciplines can learn of the function of those from different disciplines and about their problems and solutions. One important result of this co-ordination of care is that when a patient meets several carers there should be no contradictions in what she hears them say.

Clinical/organizational meetings

In recent years, because of the problems of organization of the team and communication within it, meetings in many practices have been dominated by operational topics rather than truly clinical ones. This has been particularly so in the run-up to implementation of the 'new GP contract', and no doubt will continue until the White Paper 'turbulence' has subsided. This is unfortunate, since the patients' clinical problems should surely be the most important items for discussion on any practice agenda. Clinical meetings must be accorded priority as soon as possible. These meetings should be attended by all the doctors and their trainees and medical students, fortified by the expertise of other members of the team relevant to the particular clinical subject. Accordingly, the practice nurses will frequently be present, but when paediatric or obstetric problems are being discussed health-visitor, midwife, and even social workers could well become involved. In my own practice we aim to have two clinical-meeting working-lunches per month. They have been recognized by the Regional Adviser as qualifying for the Postgraduate Educational Allowance. The informal appointment of a practice clinical tutor to organize the programme, run the meetings, ensure their academic rigour, and co-ordinate participants' evaluation later is vital.

Protocol meetings

As the care in the practice increasingly devolves onto 'clinics', it is important that protocols for the care of 'clinic illnesses' are established. The practice nurse undertakes most of the work and will find her medical knowledge stretched. The doctors' share in the care of these chronic illnesses will decrease.[4] From the protocol meetings can emerge mini-clinics for pre-conception counselling, diabetes, vascular disease, new patients, geriatrics, menopause and hormone-replacement therapy, asthma, psoriasis, and so on. Some of these protocols are described in Chapter 4. Their overriding aim is to ensure a more comprehensive and detailed care of patients with these conditions.

Business meetings

When the financial welfare of the practice is under scrutiny, business meetings are needed at which the accountant will attend and the practice manager will play an important role. Ideally, the accountant should be one who has had experience in practice accounting and an interest in the medical field. Our own accountant was on the local Family Practitioner Committee for many years and is now chairman of our District Health Authority!

Receptionists' meeting

Lay members of the practice need a forum at which they can express their views on how the practice is, or should be, functioning. Here too they can be informed of the practice's changing methods and comment from their point of view. In many shops and other service-orientated businesses, the 'shop' closes for two hours a week for 'staff training'. There seems no reason why practices should not do this, so long as emergency telephone cover is provided. Our receptionists have a two-hour working-lunch once a fortnight.

WHO LEADS THE TEAM?

The team should function democratically, not hierarchically.[2,5] It would be invidious of the general practitioner to assume that he is the leader of the team when he is working with independent professional colleagues such as social workers, health-visitors, ministers of the church, counsellors, and so on. It is better if GPs look upon themselves as co-ordinators rather than leaders. It is the problem that the patient presents which leads the team, and those primarily responsible for that problem will, for a period, lead the team in dealing with it. Hence leadership can change from week to week as problems come and go. As an example, a counsellor providing care for an obese, impotent, 45-year-old male patient may well ask the doctor to exclude incipient or even overt diabetes. In addition, she may involve the dietitian in the reduction of his obesity and perhaps the practice nurse in a well-man clinic in order to receive advice on general fitness.

Certainly, many teams have foundered and many more never become established because of an automatic assumption by the doctors in them that they lead and that they will organize their colleagues according to their own preference.[6] As one overt example of the democracy of the team, a doctor should by no means chair all the team meetings, in particular if he is the partner longest in post!

WHO IN THE TEAM IS ULTIMATELY RESPONSIBLE?

The patient's doctor is probably ultimately responsible for the majority of care that takes place. There is no doubt that when patients perceive that errors have been made, it is to the doctor that they complain and it is the doctor that they sue. For that reason, other team members must appreciate that it is usually appropriate, particularly where matters of clinical, social, or psychological moment are being managed, that the doctor should at least have some awareness of what is going on. Although in theory this sounds a complicated problem, in day-to-day practice where communication is good and note-keeping consistent, it very rarely proves to be so.

WHO IN THE TEAM IS ACCESSIBLE?

Where personal lists operate—and this book recommends them for their efficiency (see Chapter 8)—the patient's own doctor should provide sufficient appointments so that he can see all routine appointments within a day or two and have a reasonable ability to fit in emergencies in his patients within the working day. In a recent study in my own practice, 85 per cent of the consultations were managed by the patient's own doctor, and considering that the doctor is away six weeks per annum on holiday, two weeks per annum on study leave, and works on a rota system on an approximately one-in-seven basis for evenings and weekends, the proportion of own-doctor consultations is laudably high. All members of the team should be accessible to patients and be given appropriate accommodation in order to consult (see Chapter 1).

WORKING AS A TEAM FROM THE PATIENT'S POINT OF VIEW

Patients expect team members to work together and share ideas. They realize that when health care professionals discuss problems together, the opinions that are formed will be more considered—'two heads are better than one'. They like to be able to consult other team members as an alternative to the doctor. Too many practices have all male doctors and female team members are particularly appreciated.

REFERENCES

1. Marsh, G. N. and Thornham, J. R. (1980). Changing to A4 folders and updating records in a 'busy' general practice'. *British Medical Journal*, **281**, 215–17.

2. Marsh, G. and Kaim-Caudle, P. (1976). *Team Care in General Practice*. London: Croom Helm.
3. Kaim-Caudle, P. R. and Marsh, G. N. (1975). Patient satisfaction survey in general practice. *British Medical Journal*, **1**, 262–4.
4. Hasler, J. and Schofield, T. (eds.) (1990). *Continuing care: the management of chronic disease*, 2nd edn. Oxford: OUP.
5. Greig, D. N. H. (1988). *Team work in general practice*. Tunbridge Wells: Castle House.
6. Wilkin, D. Hallam, L., Leavey, R., and Metcalfe, D. (1987). *Anatomy of urban general practice*. London: Tavistock.

3. Home visits

Home visiting is the jewel in the crown of British general practice.[1] Its volume sets British practices apart from practices in other English-speaking countries in the world. The British patient cherishes her doctor coming to her own home when she considers she is sufficiently sick for it to be inappropriate to go to the surgery. In recent years complaints about doctors being reluctant to visit have become increasingly strident.

Home visiting is the most time-wasting exercise in general practice. Where it is overdone, either because the doctor has not educated his patients sufficiently about the need for surgery attendance, or where patients are making inappropriate demands for home visits, the resultant shortage of time and even sheer exhaustion can make the doctor's life miserable.

It is the task of this chapter to reconcile the contradictory statements in the above two paragraphs.

Most doctors find that they can do about four visits per hour, including travelling time, in urban settings; considerably fewer in less-densely populated areas. As the number of home visits falls, the time per visit obviously increases since the travelling time for each one becomes dispro-portionately greater. On the other hand, many doctors see ten patients per hour in the surgery. So in terms of time, the cost-effectiveness of home visits is poor.

The obligation on general practitioners to visit patients in their homes when necessary has been embodied in the National Health Service Acts. However, Kenneth Robinson, a former Minister of Health, stated categor-ically that it was the doctor's decision, based on information received about the request, as to whether a home visit was necessary. It follows, of course, that if the doctor decides wrongly and harm comes to the patient as a result of not visiting, then the doctor is culpable; as a result he will have problems, most importantly with his own conscience, but possibly also with his Family Health Services Authority (formerly FPC) and ultimately the General Medical Council. Recently, the GMC has become less rigid about the interpretation of 'failure to visit', and with greater accessibility of patients to practices (see later) and a greater awareness of the abuse of requests for home visits, failure to visit has become a less frequent cause for investigation.

DATA ON HOME VISITING

Two major studies of home visiting in the northern region of England produced seminal papers in the *British Medical Journal*, the first in 1972 and the second in 1983.[2,3]Approximately 200 general practitioners provided data for both these studies, and it is probable that the picture presented, and the changes shown across the years, are fairly representative of many areas of Great Britain. In 1969 the average general practitioner in northern England did 9.1 home visits per day (Mondays to Fridays) and in 1980 he was doing 5.4: a reduction of 41 per cent. New visits—that is, visits requested by patients—had fallen by 31 per cent, from 4.5 to 3.1 per day. Repeat visits generated by the doctor had fallen by 57 per cent, from 2.8 to 1.2, and chronic visits—that is, generated by the doctor but to patients with chronic continuing disease—had fallen by 39 per cent, from 1.8 to 1.1. The greatest change was a reduction of 80 per cent in visits to babies (under 1 year old). Contrarily, for the over-65s there was an actual rise of 16 per cent for new requested visits. In addition, the over-65s had a relatively small reduction of only 24 per cent for repeat visits (chronics included). Also, 34 per cent of all visits, and 68 per cent of repeat visits, were made to patients over 65 (about 12 per cent of the population). The relatively high visiting-rate for the elderly was associated with a significant number of visits for dementia, and this was the only clinical area where visiting had increased. For other clinical conditions, the biggest change was visiting for respiratory infections, which fell by over 50 per cent. In both the 1969 and 1980 studies, doctors reckoned that, even allowing for the social vicissitudes of the patients, about 25 per cent of the visits could have come to the surgery. There was patently a continuing need for education of both patient and doctor.

The fall in visits was ascribed to various factors. First, in response to patient education, usually on a one-to-one basis by doctors and other members of the team, supported by a certain amount of Government propaganda, it has increasingly become the conventional wisdom that when sick you go to see the doctor at his surgery. Secondly, there is greater availability of transport, in particular rising car-ownership. The two-car family has become more common, making it very easy for mothers in such families to bring their children to the surgery, no matter what their illness. Although the centralization of surgeries associated with the formation of large group-practices militates against the geographical proximity of patients, the majority of these large centres have been sited near bus stops, hence facilitating access. Thirdly, the government's relaxation of rules for sickness certification, including 'do-it-yourself' certificates for short-term illness, has also lessened the need for the visiting of the 'short-term' sick at home.

That visiting has not fallen more is partly ascribed to the higher proportion of elderly in the population, coupled with their increasing expectations in a more sophisticated, caring, and wealthy society. In addition, there has been poor use of the nurses in the primary health-care team, evidenced by the fact that in 1969 only in 14.8 per cent of visits was the nurse asked to go on a subsequent occasion, and in 1980 this percentage had fallen to 6.7 per cent. It seems that the team is not being well used.

Variation in visiting rates

But probably the most interesting statistic, and the one most relevant to this book, was the variation in home visits between one practice and another. A quarter of practices were doing four times the number of visits of the quarter at the other extreme. This applied to practices working almost side by side in the same towns or the same rural areas! But just as importantly, the doctor-to-doctor variation in numbers of visits was even greater than the practice-to-practice variations. Again this applied where doctors were working in the same areas with the same type of patients. Even within the same practice there were variations of five, six, and seven times between one partner and another, despite each partner having the same age and social class of patients.

HOW DO WE REDUCE VISITING?

So how do we reduce visiting, save time and effort, and become accordingly more efficient? Considerable reductions can flow from further promulgating the reasons given above for the fall in visiting between 1969 and 1972. Remember that 25 per cent of visits were thought to be unnecessary in 1969, yet despite a reduction of 40 per cent by 1972, 25 per cent were still thought to be unnecessary. Clearly there is still room for further reductions.

Patient education

Practice policy on home visits should be discussed at the team meetings (most appropriately at the house committee—see Chapter 2), where all members of the team involved in visiting can contribute. It is important that all team members share the same aims; indeed, most doctors find that community nurses are just as irritated by unnecessary visits to patients' homes as they are. It must become the conventional wisdom of the practice team—and then be passed on to the patients—that if people, particularly the elderly chronic sick, leave home for other reasons (for example, to visit the hairdressers, pick up their pension, or go to church), then it is not unreasonable for them to come to the surgery. Patients with transport available (including helpful relatives and neighbours) should certainly be expected to use it or have someone drive them to the surgery. The erroneous 'wisdom' that children with temperatures should not be taken out of the house should be corrected—cooling down by exposure to fresh air can be therapeutic.

Trained receptionists

The receptionists in particular must know that the team's aim is to get people to come to the surgery for their care. They must know the practice policy on visiting with regard to minor illnesses such as chicken-pox and influenza. In my own practice there was success in the recent epidemic when requests for visits for influenza were declined, except for the elderly, the chronic sick, babies, and the socially deprived. The practice reception- ists reinforced the Department of Health's instructions on the treatment of influenza and, from time to time with patients who wished, offered to have the doctor telephone back. With this attitude to 'the 'flu', our practice was not unduly burdened.

If a particular receptionist takes requests for home visits each morning between 8.30 a.m. and 10.00 a.m. she can become relatively expert in this area. Indeed, she will get to know the chronic sick, especially the house- bound, and be a familiar voice on the telephone to them. She will be adept at proffering alternatives to those requesting home visits. The following 'aids' are helpful:

(1) to be able to offer quick surgery appointments that day and preferably that morning—particularly helpful for children with earache, patients with abdominal pain, patients acutely anxious, and so on;

(2) proffering some other member of the team as an alternative to the doctor; for example, offering a community nurse to visit a patient just out of hospital: frequently their skills are more appropriate, since the major need could well be for nursing, dressings, supervision of convalescence, and the like;

(3) taking the patient's phone-number so that the doctor can telephone at the end of the morning surgery: armed with the patient's notes he can talk to her and decide whether a home visit is really necessary (see Chapter 13).

If, despite all the above efforts, doctors and nurses find themselves doing a home visit which is patently unreasonable, then when all the necessary care and attention has been given they can indicate to the patient—without causing offence—that a surgery attendance, or even self care, would have been appropriate. The major reason for bothering to counsel people in this way is the hope that on subsequent occasions they will act more appropriately.

Practice boundaries

The further away patients live from the surgery, the more likely they are to request home visits. This is particularly so where they have no transport of their own, and even more so if they have to change buses. Hence there is often a disproportionate amount of time spent visiting a small number of patients living far away from the surgery. In our own practice in the late 1960s we analysed where our patients lived and removed 600 of them from the practice list who lived in areas which were difficult to reach. These 600 patients were on the whole extremely understanding—including many of those who had used the practice for years—and they settled rapidly into new practices nearer their own homes. The doctors of those practices were initially irritated—it was at a time when work-load was high, practices ill-organized, and teams virtually non-existent—and some of them removed patients from their practices who lived near our surgery. Hence our patient numbers were restored, but by people who could come to the surgery easily. There is no doubt that a defined practice boundary, orientating particularly on convenient access for patients via bus-routes and easy roads, is enormously important. It does not seem beyond the bounds of possibility for practices in urban areas to get together and 'trade patients' in order to make their practice boundaries tighter. Having defined a practice boundary, it is extremely important that all partners subscribe to it, and 'favourite' patients, long-known faces, and familiar friends be obliged to leave the practice if they move across it. Practice boundaries can be reassessed from time to time if roads or bus-services change, or if new surgery premises open up in areas distant from your own surgery where you have patients.

If more sick patients are to come to the surgery, it is important that there should be a handicapped-parking area provided near the entrance and, once inside, that corridors and consulting-room doors should be adequate for wheelchair access and that there should be a toilet with facilities for handicapped people.

Preventative measures

As immunization-rates for measles and pertussis rise towards the 'herd immunity' levels of about 90 per cent—largely as a result of the 'new contract's' method of payment (!)—these diseases, which were traditionally visited at home, will disappear. By accurate recall systems for influenza vaccination of the chronic sick with illnesses such as chronic bronchitis, congestive heart failure, diabetes, and so on, the effect of epidemics will be minimized and the associated high visiting work-load of these vulnerable patients will be reduced.

Use of the team

Remember that after only 14.8 per cent of visits in 1969 was a community nurse asked to do a follow-up visit. This figure had fallen to 6.7 per cent in 1980. Team care seemed to be at a low ebb.

Acute new visits

Since the community nurses are not 'nurse-practitioners', and accordingly do not establish new diagnoses (at least officially!), their role in responding to requests for acute new visits is limited (see Chapter 1). However, with the receptionists trained to collect information on the telephone, community nurses can follow up hospital discharges and, from time to time, visit in place of the doctor to confirm a diagnosis of a previous acute illness which is recorded in the notes (for example, recurrent back strain). Occasionally the doctor can send the nurse after a telephone consultation, so that she can confirm the diagnosis that he has made. Although initially in our own practice we employed our own practice nurse to do visits of this type, the community nurses have now absorbed this into their remit.[4,5] The numbers are small. With their narrower spectrum, midwives are probably better able to do new visits and make diagnoses because of their expertise in one particular area.

Repeat visits in acute episodes

It was in this type of visit that the greatest reduction took place between 1969 and 1980—a fall of 57 per cent—and it is probably in this area where the greatest doctor-to-doctor variation takes place, yet these repeat visits are almost totally under the control of the doctor himself. Such visits should be clinically necessary and in need of the doctor's physical examination and therapeutic expertise. For the purpose of routine, ongoing assessment of illness nurses are totally appropriate—they do this constantly for hospital in-patients as part of their standard care. In the paediatric field, health-visitors can assess the continuing care and improvement of sick children, as can midwives in the antenatal or puerperal period. Some doctors now use the telephone to assess patients' progress rather than paying repeat visits. Importantly, part of the education taking place around any acute illness is an outline of its course: the anticipated response to therapy and how the illness and recovery should progress. If this is done well, the responsibility for recall can mostly be left to the patients themselves.

Chronic disease

Despite the increase in the age of the population, there was a 39 per cent reduction in doctor-initiated visits to the chronically ill between 1969 and 1980. During that time the chronic sick had received increasing provision in other ways. Home-helps had increased, warden-supervised accommodation was more common, and increasingly available were day hospitals, day centres, clubs, and workshops. All this made the 'social' visit by the general practitioner each month less important than it used to be. Some of the elderly sick are now too busy and can't 'wait in' for their monthly visit!

After visits to the chronic sick, doctors should ask themselves the following questions:

(a) was the visit clinically or diagnostically interesting?

(b) was it therapeutically valuable?

(c) could someone else have done it?

(d) does this patient leave home for other purposes (hairdressers and so on)?

(e) could the communication have been made on the telephone?

It is now becoming commonplace for the community nursing sister and the doctor to share the care of the chronic house-bound sick, the nurse perhaps going once a month for two months, and the doctor going on the third month. The nurse's popularity with the chronic house-bound sick is extremely high and her visits are inordinately welcome.

Recently, elderly-care visitors (ECVs) have visited all patients in my practice over the age of 75; a system now embodied in the 'new contract' for general practitioners. At this visit the ECV assesses the patient's overall care, including their psycho-social needs. Indeed, in chronically sick, house-bound patients with multiple general problems I have asked the ECV to analyse these and organize appropriate provisions. Such home visits have been extremely well received by the elderly, and the work is not done by the doctor.

The psycho-geriatric nurse fairly recently attached to our practice has undertaken a great deal of the day-to-day care of elderly psychotic and demented patients (see Chapter 1). Most of them, by virtue of their conditions, are visited at home. In the 1980 survey, the 16 per cent increase in elderly visiting was largely attributed to the demented; the attached psycho-geriatric nurse has now mitigated that problem.

Traditionally, the community psychiatric nurse has cared for the chronic psychotics in the community—schizophrenics, agoraphobes, and so on— usually visiting them at home. This is still an important role but she is well able to work with acute problems too (see Chapter 1). Many of them she can follow up and supervise, and our nurse seems particularly happy to visit patients in their own home for this.

MacMillan nurses, specially trained in the care of the dying, can share care with and provide expertise for the doctor. Their work is done almost entirely by visiting patients in their own homes.

'Stoma' nurses have recently provided an expertise for patients with various types of 'ostomy' and carry out their work in patients' homes. Their up-to-date knowledge contrasts with that of confused or out-of-date doctors.

Late and out-of-hours calls

After 10.00 a.m. the doctor should speak to all requests for home visits for that day, with the clinical record in front of him. He can do this either immediately, or can ring the patient back. Only in cases which the receptionist considered grave, and where the doctor was out of the surgery, would the call be accepted and the doctor 'bleeped' to go immediately. The great majority of these requests for late visits can be converted, either to telephone advice or to patients or relatives collecting an interim prescription. Alternatively, although the receptionists find it difficult to persuade such patients to come to the surgery, the doctor finds it relatively easy.

For out-of-hours calls, the tape-recording indicating which doctor is on duty and providing his phone-number says that his number should be 'rung for advice about urgent medical problems'. There is no implication in this message that the doctor will visit. Accordingly, as many as half our callers now say on speaking to the doctor that they 'just want some advice' or 'can you advise me what to do'. This puts the responsibility for visiting plainly on the doctor's shoulders, and from the history that he can take on the telephone he can decide whether to go. In a recent survey from my practice, only 40 per cent of telephone calls between 6.00 p.m. and 8.00 p.m. received a visit, and after analysis of records later no patients had come to harm.[6] An increasing number of practices now seem to be working in this way.[7,8]

Personal visiting

In the early 1960s I was doing about eighteen visits per day, in the early 1970s ten per day, and in the early 1980s three or four per day. Now in the 1990s I do an average of two or three visits per day, but in order to reduce the time per visit spent travelling I try to do most of them on one particular morning in the week. Hence on other days I can leave my car in the garage and walk to work, and usually do not have to return and get it out.

Overall work-load

Despite the fall in home visiting shown in the two studies, it was surprising to note that there was also a concomitant 23 per cent reduction in surgery consultations. Patently the total volume of work had fallen. Presumably this cannot continue, and the provision of more surgeries will ultimately become (or has already become) necessary. Certainly all the extra clinics for preventative care, geriatric surveillance, developmental paediatrics, and minor-ops sessions, necessitated under the terms of the 'new contract', have made the volume of surgery work rise. Likewise, the implications of the White Paper, with the devolvement of much hospital out-patient follow-up care on to general practice, will necessitate more time being needed in the surgery. To be able to fulfil this new-style service, home visiting will have to be curtailed in the ways I have suggested.

RESULTS OF LESS VISITING

As a result of doing fewer visits, doctors are less tired and can do more surgeries, teach, research, and organize and supervise preventative care. The smaller number of visits remaining are done more joyfully and provide a pleasant break from continuing 'office' involvement. Because they have time available, doctors can carry out more visits to seriously ill patients, for example, to a myocardial infarction being treated at home or to a severe exacerbation of asthma, or to the dying. The gravely ill can be seen two or three times in the same day where neceasary. Repeat visits can be made to assess problematical cases, such as an abdominal pain which might be appendicitis. Because of this intensive home care of such 'problem' patients, the referral-rate to hospital falls; 'budget' economies are made. Doctors can also provide more prompt reaction to true emergency calls. Less chronic visiting becomes more clinically rewarding, and new diagnoses should not be missed—always a problem when ritual monthly visits were common.

HOME VISITS FROM THE PATIENT'S POINT OF VIEW

Patients are increasingly aware that the cherished home visit is becoming a luxury, and is time-consuming for the doctor. Because of their increasing mobility, two-car ownership, and so on (see earlier), many more patients now seem prepared to attend surgery so long as that attendance is at a time convenient to them and ultimately clinically worthwhile. Indeed, it is often apparent to them that more comprehensive care can be provided at the surgery than they can receive in their own homes. Immediate availability of a computerized record, various team members, and appropriate instruments are notably lacking in the patient's bedroom. Not infrequently patients now use taxis to come to the surgery—the response of a more affluent society.

Many practices, however, have a core of socially deprived families, and trained receptionists must be aware of their special needs. This will include acquiescing more readily to requests for home visits because of the psychosocial constraints that many of these families are obliged to tolerate.

Patients will be aware that if the doctor's total visiting-load is reduced he will be able to provide more home-care for those truly needing it (the critically ill, the dying, and so on), and will also be more instantly available to sudden life-threatening emergencies.

Follow-up visits by nurses are uniformly acceptable by patients. My patient-satisfaction research, even in the early days of this 'consultative' nurse visiting, found that only 4 per cent of patients who had received a follow-up visit from a nurse felt that this was inappropriate.[9] Only 2 per cent lacked confidence in the nurse reporting new problems to the doctor or in the doctor taking the necessary action. At that time nurses were also used for new visits, but in about 25 per cent of such visits the patients felt that they had problems with which the nurses could not cope. Accordingly, new visits have been minimized (see above). For visits to chronic housebound patients, two-thirds of them thought that the doctor and the nurse did the same job when they saw them! Again, there was high satisfaction with nurse-care and confidence that nurse and doctor were working together and new problems would be noted. The patient's perception of doctor and nurse working as a team seems all-important.

REFERENCES

1. Gray, D. J. P. (1978). Feeling ill at home. *Journal of the Royal College of General Practitioners*, **28**, 6–17.
2. Marsh, G. N., McNay, R. A., and Whewell, J. (1972). Survey of home visiting by general practitioners in north-east England. *British Medical Journal*, **1**, 487–92.
   3. Whewell, J., Marsh, G. N., and McNay, R. A. (1983). Changing patterns of home visiting in the north of England. *British Medical Journal*, **286**, 1259–61.
4. Marsh, G. N. (1969). Visiting nurse—analysis of one year's work. *British Medical Journal*, **4**, 42–4.
5. Marsh, G. N. (1967). Group practice nurse: an analysis and comment on six months' work. *British Medical Journal*, **1**, 489–91.
6. Marsh, G. N., Horne, R. A., and Channing, D. M. (1987). A study of

telephone advice in managing out-of-hours calls. *Journal of the Royal College of General Practitioners*, **37**, 301–4.
7. Knox, J. D. E. (1989). *On-call: out-of-hours telephone calls and home visits*. Oxford University Press.
8. Allsop, J. and May, A. (1985). *Telephone access to GPs in the UK: a study of London*. King Edward's Hospital Fund, London.
9. Marsh, G. N. and Kaim-Caudle, P. (1976). *Team Care in General Practice.*, Croom Helm, London.

4. The efficient management of clinical conditions

If the doctor establishes the correct diagnosis and the appropriate therapy, people will get better promptly; clearly this is efficient care. Hence the established, experienced, clinically confident, well-trained, well-refreshed general practitioner is more likely to carry out his work efficiently than his 'opposite' counterpart, and because his patients are cured, they will not require any follow-up nor will they feel it necessary to re-consult.

MINIMIZING RETURN CONSULTATIONS

One of the most fundamental aspects of any consultation is the education of the patient about her illness, the therapy, and about its progress to recovery.[1,2] If the doctor takes the time at this first consultation to make an accurate diagnosis, and considers the therapy carefully and correctly, he can then spell out fairly definitely the course of the illness and the time it will take to get better. So the patient leaves, probably without any need to make a further appointment. Patently, if the progress the doctor has outlined does not materialize, she is free to make a further appointment: all part of the health education of the first consultation. Perhaps the most important element in this type of care is the need to spell out to the patient the course of the illness and the time it will take. Obviously, for long illnesses or those in which progress cannot be assessed by the patients themselves, it may well be appropriate to invite them to make a return appointment. But for the many conditions which are not serious and are expected to resolve in a few weeks, return appointments can be avoided. The proportion of patient-initiated to doctor-initiated consultations in practices varies enormously, and doctors who have a large proportion of the latter will almost certainly have a higher work-load. By following the steps spelled out above follow-up work-load can be reduced.

Fortifying the doctor's account of how the illness will progress, and facilitated by good date-ordered continuing records, be they manual or on computer screens, will be the amazing fact that most patients have had most of their illnesses before (see Chapter 10). Bronchitics have had episodes of bronchitis; catarrhal children have had otitis media and tonsillitis; adolescents have had ingrown toe-nails; cervical spondylitics will have had neck pain; depressives will have had depression; women of child-bearing age will have had thrush and cystitis; osteo-arthritics will have had joint pain; dyspeptics will have had indigestion. The patients themselves will be well aware of the prognosis, plus the treatment and its effectiveness, and the doctor can, by recap on previous experience, improve the accuracy of his care. Thus the doctor should not need to initiate many follow-up consultations. It can be left to the patient to reconsult if the progress is not as projected, or is dissimilar to the previous successful outcome.

MINIMIZING INVESTIGATION

There is great variation in the amount of investigation that individual doctors carry out on their patients.[3] On the whole, over-investigation of illness tends to produce more work, so from a cost-effective point of view there is credit in minimizing investigations as much as possible. Ann Cartwright has suggested that 'quality' in general practice means non-investigation of symptoms that will clear up quickly and spontaneously, as well as adequate investigations of conditions which need it.[4] When investigations are carried out, this means more work for receptionists, nurses, and the whole team, as well as for the doctor in that frequently they require further consultation and discussion. To allow illnesses of a self-limiting type to run their course—'tincture of time'—without over-investigation, certainly reduces the hassle of care, and both patients' and doctors' over-involvement. Even if investigations are discussed on the telephone or via receptionists, there is work involved (see Chapter 3). So keep to minimal and appropriate investigations only; on balance this decreases the volume of the job, not to mention minimizing costs for fund-holding practices.

EMPIRICAL TREATMENT

It was always considered clinically acceptable to carry out therapeutic trials of TNT to help establish a diagnosis of angina. By the same token, it seems not unreasonable—so long as patients are well selected and appropriately examined—to carry out other empirical treatments. The use of a Salbutamol inhaler for possible bronchospasm, of Cimetidine for gastric problems, and tricyclic drugs for depression are further examples.[5] Such empirical treatment is now accepted by medical specialists.

MINIMAL HOSPITAL REFERRAL

The referral-rate to hospital specialists varies greatly from one doctor to another.[6,7] It is debatable whether caring for patients oneself and with the team, rather than referring them to hospital, increases or decreases work-load. On the whole, work probably increases if more serious clinical problems are managed in the setting of the community, but not as much as would appear at first sight. Patients are frequently over-investigated in hospital, then return to their homes with continuing problems to be evaluated, so that work for the general practitioner continues. The more circumscribed and concise care given by the GP leaves less to be 'sorted out'. It should be possible to use consultants more on the telephone regarding clinical problems rather than actually referring the patients in person. 'I just want to pick your brains about . . .'—the beginning of a telephone consultation from a concerned GP to a consultant might make referral unnecessary. As special clinics develop in practices (see later) and one partner becomes 'expert' at a particular disease (diabetes, for example), this partner could refine telephone contact with a relevant specialist colleague. In this way, out-patient referral—and certainly follow-up—could be minimized.[8]

PROTOCOLS OF CARE

Many clinical illnesses lend themselves to a check-list of measurements. When these measurements are made, then the illness is appropriately assessed and its ongoing care can be organized and scheduled. Thus emerges the concept of 'protocol care'. Consciously or unconsciously, in ordinary surgery attendances doctors use mental protocols when consider-ing the investigation and therapy of illnesses such as diabetes, angina, and hypertension. For nursing staff, whose breadth of knowledge is not as wide as the doctor's, protocols are even more important. The best-known example of protocol care is the midwife's antenatal care: checking of certain parameters—weight, blood-pressure, urine, fundal height—at each attend-ance, and extra parameters at specified times—haemoglobin and blood glucose at eight weeks and thirty weeks, and so on. Nursing staff, in my experience, enjoy working to protocols. They do it better than doctors.

There now follows a description of ten examples to illustrate the general principles of protocol care. None of them are written in pillars of stone, all of them are incomplete and can be varied according to individual practice situations or individual patients; they will all be modified as clinical knowledge changes. Most importantly, they will serve as a spring-board to others. Read what follows, then adopt them or make your own.

1. Patients discharged from hospital post-operatively

It is important to anticipate the patient's discharge from hospital prior to her actually going in. Hence instructions to people being admitted for major surgery, such as cholecystectomy, mastectomy, or major gastro-intestinal surgery are that when they have returned from hospital they should 'potter about at home a bit' and then come and see their doctor. This erases doubt from the patient's mind about whether to request a home visit on return from hospital as well as giving a general guide-line. Many patients may have dressings, and they could be told that if there are problems with the dressing or the wound in some way, then an appropriate home visit could be requested from the community nurse. Indeed, many hospitals organize community nurses to visit without involving their doctors. Similarly, if patients are being sent into hospital as an emergency, such as appendicitis, incomplete abortion, or perforated duodenal ulcer, again they or their relatives can be advised at that time about convalescence on return home and and when to see their own doctor again. Anticipatory planning (a protocol) used in this way prevents unnecessary home visits.

For patients who are receiving specialist care, such as the care of a major eye problem, somewhat inconsequential surgery consultations can be avoided by suggesting that their continuing care 'can be left to the experts at the hospital'. A caveat that 'if there are any problems that crop up in the intervals' then patients can come and see their own doctor leaves the door open without the patient feeling the necessity always to be walking through it!

2. Thyroid deficiency

Once the diagnosis has been established and the correct dose achieved, patients taking Thyroxin for thyroid deficiency remain extremely well. Amongst GP colleagues there is great debate as to whether these patients do need to be seen routinely for a 'thyroid check', and certainly there is great doubt amongst endocrinologists as to whether patients feeling well on Thyroxin maintenance actually do need to have blood taken for a TSH estimation.[9] My practice is to tell the patients to get repeat prescriptions; if they do not feel completely well then by all means request a TSH estimation via the receptionist; they can check the result with them—if it is normal then their Thyroxin is being effective. I also take the opportunity during intercurrent illnesses—sprained ankles, skin problems, and the like—to mention their thyroid and ask about general energy and feeling of well-being at that time.

3. Pernicious anaemia

There is considerable evidence from the volume of Vitamin B12 used in Great Britain that large numbers of patients are receiving B12 who do not have a deficiency, and even those who do are having their injections too frequently.[10] Correct therapy for pernicious anaemia at the appropriate intervals—three-monthly for most patients—coupled with a reassessment of the diagnostic accuracy of all those routinely having B12, would certainly reduce its use and, coincidentally, costs. It would also reduce doctors' and nurses' work considerably. But for those correctly diagnosed and established on three-monthly injections, like those with thyroid deficiency, it would seem that if they feel well and see the nurse for their injections, then nothing more needs to be done. Lethargy or lack of well-being, would indicate to the nurse that she should take some blood to check any inappropriate response to therapy.

4. Epilepsy

The main indicator that all is well with the medication of epileptic patients is that they are having no fits. Their medication should also be simple—preferably one drug only.[11,12] It is probably wise for them to have medication blood-levels measured perhaps once a year, even though they remain fit-free, since sometimes these are unnecessarily high, hence increasing the risk of side-effects, and in the younger age-groups the blood-level can fall below the therapeutic range as they increase in size. I normally tell all my adult epileptic patients to have an annual blood-test. They can check the result with the receptionists, and if they are not having fits and feel well there is no need to re-consult. As with other illnesses above, I ask about their epilepsy when I see them for other intercurrent illnesses. All my epileptics are instructed as to when and whether they might try to reduce medication when they have been fit-free for a specified period of time, but I usually insist that they see me before a reduction programme takes place, since supervision is necessary and careful instructions are to be followed at this time.

5. Asthma

In the above illnesses, the nurse's involvement has been relatively minor: mostly just taking blood, giving injections, and querying general well-being. For the asthmatic once diagnosed, however, there is a great deal of follow-up that nurses can do, and indeed practice nurses are now beginning to run formal asthma clinics, both for children and young adults as well as for maturity-onset asthmatics.[13] Once appropriately investigated and diagnosed, and treatment established, nurses can continue to see asthmatic patients, write up their continuing care in their record, or enter it on their computer screen. They are particularly valuable for checking the new starter's inhaler technique and identifying provocation factors, as well as explaining the condition and providing leaflets. They also measure routinely peak-flow and record this on the notes. They can teach patients how to measure their own peak-flow and how to modify their treatment in response to readings. They can offer patients appropriate repeat appointments for continuing supervision. Where problems occur, or therapy is not proving effective, then the GP can be involved. If the practice runs a patient asthma group—popular and well attended in my own practice—the nurse can attend in order to discuss asthma with patients as a group and also show films or give short lectures. Several hundred nurses have attended the Asthma Society Training Centre in Stratford-upon-Avon for courses on the care of asthma.[14] Drug firms are very prepared to back up asthma clinics in surgeries, and in particular help nurses to improve their expertise.

Many general practitioners find the care of asthma an extremely time-consuming affair, and the sharing of care with nurses, as described above, certainly reduces this. I commend it to you.

6. Diabetes

The establishment of mini-clinics, particularly for maturity onset diabetics, has been one of the major 'growth areas' in general practice in recent years.[15,16,17] That most of the work can be done by nurses is becoming increasingly apparent.[15,17] In some regions nurse facilitators have been appointed to go to practices without clinics and help establish them.[18]

The maturity-onset diabetic is usually diagnosed by her GP in his surgery. At that consultation the patient can be given an introductory leaflet spelling out the major dietary restrictions prior to seeing the dietitian. The patient then attends, ideally within a week, the practice diabetic clinic run jointly by the nurse and the dietitian. The dietitian refines the introductory dietary advice and arranges a follow-up. The nurse does an overall assessment of the patient, including height/weight ratio, smoking history, alcohol-intake assessment, family history of diabetes, symptoms prior to diagnosis, measurement of blood-pressure, advice about attending the optician annually, inspection of feet and explanation of foot-care and the use of the chiropodist, checking peripheral pulses, reflexes, and vibration sense, and instructing patients on testing urine for sugar, and also carries out a check for albumen. The patient is told to carry out several urine tests prior to the next appointment. She is also advised about applying for free prescriptions, informing her driving-insurance company and the DVLC in Swansea, and advised to join the British Diabetic Association. Leaflets and pamphlets can be made available. If blood has not been taken, this can be done also. The nurse can offer continued support on the telephone in the interim between then and the next visit. Newly diagnosed patients do require frequent appointments until they become confident in managing their diabetes.

Once diagnosed and assessed comprehensively in this way, non-insulin dependent diabetics can be seen every six months.

Insulin-dependent diabetics, once stabilized, can also have their interim care carried out at the nurse diabetic clinic, usually by three-monthly visits.

At subsequent appointments, diabetic patients see the dietitian and the nurse will check weight, enquire about general well-being, test urine for protein, review medication, reassess smoking and drinking habits, check blood-pressure, and, at least annually, inspect feet, check peripheral pulses, reflexes and sensation, check regular attendance at optician and arrange fundoscopy with doctor if necessary.

It is probably advisable for the nurse to take blood for urea, elctrolytes, full blood-count, fructosamine and triglycerides and cholesterol approximately every year.

Patently, any problems with the management of the diabetes can be referred to the doctor who 'shadows' this diabetic clinic; any other medical problems can be referred to the patient's GP.

It is estimated that a national screening programme for diabetes, including inspection of retinas for early diabetic retinopathy could possibly prevent about 260 new cases of blindness in diabetics in Great Britain under the age of 70 each year.[19]

7. Vascular clinic

In my own practice, we use the term vascular clinic to include the follow-up of patients with various forms of pathology in the cardio-vascular and cerebro-vascular systems. This therefore includes patients with hypertension, angina, and those recovering from myocardial infarction and strokes. The doctor will have done a great deal of care for these patients in the acute episode or around the newly established diagnosis. These are serious illnesses and patients expect this. The variations in the severity of the illnesses, not to mention variation in type of patient, are certainly sufficiently problematic to tax the full clinical expertise of a doctor. It is when they settle into the ongoing routine care that the vascular clinic comes into its own, where nurses working to protocols can continue assessment.

Hypertensives

The recently diagnosed hypertensive may have been suspected at an attendance at a well-man or well-woman clinic, or have been detected opportunistically by his own doctor at a surgery attendance (see Chapter 7). It is first of all important to estimate the blood-pressure with the appropriate cuff-width at different times of day to establish the diagnosis.[20] The nurse will then take blood for profile and serum lipids. After this initial assessment the patient can then return to their own doctor for advice regarding therapy, including possible medication. Once the hypertension is controlled, the patient can then return to the vascular clinic for continuing care. Depending on the degree of hypertension, and working to a record-sheet profile or vascular clinic computer screen, the nurse will check pulse, blood-pressure, weight, and give advice on diet, routines regarding exercise, smoking, alcohol, as well as side-effects of medication and overall progress.

Post myocardial infarction/angina, and so on

The protocol for these illnesses is much the same as for hypertension. There is a great deal of 'literature' on these conditions, much of it of excellent quality and produced by drug firms, and this can be given to patients and discussed with them. The frequency of follow-up will vary from patient to patient, and obviously those with angina who are having attacks at perhaps more than weekly intervals will need to be followed up every two months or so, whereas those who have merely a past history of angina and are currently not having problems may need to be seen only once a year.

Acute cardiovascular or cerebrovascular illnesses at home

For many excellent reasons, not all patients with a stroke or a coronary are admitted to hospital, and general practitioners will undertake their care at home.[21–24] The community nurses are well able to share the acute management of such patients, including even two or three visits per day for the first few days in order to check blood-pressure, assess the patient's overall condition, oversee medication, support relatives, and arrange social supports—all this interwoven with the doctor's visiting. Nurses will also take appropriate blood-tests for cardiac enzymes and glucose, and carry out ECGs. Nurse and doctor working together can reduce each other's individual work-load and yet achieve a more intensive care of very sick patients in their own homes.

8. Vaginal discharges

Many general practitioners, given the known patient and good records, treat women with vaginal discharge empirically without examination.[25,26] Perhaps the best example would be a recurrence of a monilial infection after a course of antibiotics. Many women, however, need examination and high-vaginal swab-taking, and this can be carried out by the nurse who can summon the doctor to do a bi-manual examination if that has not been done recently, and either the nurse or doctor consider it appropriate. The nurse can similarly take a cervical smear if it is due, or it might be helpful in diagnosis. When the nurse has received the result of the tests she can ask the doctor to write the appropriate prescription and then follow-up the patient. My experience is that once this routine has been instituted, patients with recurrence of vaginal discharge often go directly to the nurse for any recurrence. As well as doing appropriate tests and arranging medication, the nurse can also give out all the health-education material that she has about genito-urinary problems, advise about sexual behaviour, bathing, underwear, general hygiene, and so on. It is in this area, and for these particular conditions, that the nurse is much better able to treat patients than the doctor.

9. Gastric surgery

The arrival of a patient of mine a few years ago who had had a partial gastrectomy done ten years previously, with a face as white as a sheet, short of breath, and complaining that his nails had gone a peculiar shape (Koilonychia) highlighted the need for some sort of follow-up of patients with gastrectomies. Again, such patients can attend a practice nurse at pre-ordained intervals when she can take a history, observe the general appearance of the patient, and do a full blood-count and biochemistry if she feels it appropriate. Many surgeons at hospital out-patients have post-gastrectomy clinics run by nurses, and there seems no reason why general practitioners' nurses should not do this.

10. Skin diseases

Again, once a diagnosis has been established and treatment started, continuing care can be supervised and its results inspected by nurses with training and experience.

The health-visitor can follow up napkin rashes, including carrying out swabs for fungi if appropriate. By the same token they can spend time with mothers coping with babies with infantile eczema and particularly orientate on the preventative aspects.

The community nurses frequently undertake the continuing care of hypostatic and varicose ulcers in a far more expert way than their doctor colleagues.

Warts, verrucas, ano-genital warts, and the like, once diagnosed by the doctor, can receive ongoing therapy, and supervision to cure, by practice nurses. Surely psoriasis is a skin disease waiting for a GP-clinic therapeutic protocol to be written and evaluated.

PROBLEMS ASSOCIATED WITH CLINIC PROTOCOL CARE

Initially there is a lot of work for doctor, nurse, practice manager, receptionist, and computer supervisor to do as a group in organizing and setting up the clinics outlined above. It is vital that the nurse who is going to be doing the clinic has input into the protocol and is happy with it. Nevertheless, this effort is fully rewarded as, increasingly, volumes of patients previously getting episodic, opportunistic, or even attempted pre-ordained care by their doctor, go in a more ordered way to such clinics.

One of the main problems is that initially doctors forget that the clinics exist, and they have to be reminded of them by discussing the results of the clinics from time to time at practice meetings. Also, patients can be reluctant to attend clinics, having been so conditioned to seeing their own doctor. As time goes by, however, and they appreciate the more-comprehensive care that takes place with a nurse at a clinic than with their doctor in his busy surgery, they are increasingly happy to use them. For a newly diagnosed patient, it is important that the doctor rapidly points her in the right direction; this then becomes the norm for that particular patient.

Measurements in my own practice have shown that the quality of the clinic care is much better than that given by a doctor carrying out the mental gymnastics necessary during attendances at his busy day-to-day surgery.[27] In the early attendances, it is possible that there is a certain amount of duplication of care by doctor and nurse, but as the nurse takes over this becomes increasingly uncommon; adequate records, either on paper or on screen, prevent it.

As a background to all this 'shared' care, it must be continually borne in mind that seriously ill patients, or patients with problems, are normally looked after by their doctor. Thus the detection of deterioration at the clinic is followed by rapid referral back to their doctor. Alternatively, the doctor who supervises the clinic and who has probably greater expertise than the patient's own doctor can undertake care until improvement is effected. This system leads on to the concept of 'specialoid' care within general practice; I see this as a growth-area in the next decade.

EFFICIENT MANAGEMENT OF CLINICAL CONDITIONS FROM THE PATIENT'S POINT OF VIEW

Measurements have shown not only in my own practice, that clinic protocol supervision produces better care than episodic care by the patient's own doctor.[15,28] Patients also welcome multiple access to care, many of them with chronic conditions being reticent to 'bother their doctor again'. The nurse proves a useful supportive option when they do not necessarily feel ill, but would like to discuss their condition or have it monitored in some way.

As the doctors supervising the clinics become more expert in the particular illness, it means that patients are being proffered more specialized care outside of hospitals and in the familiar setting of their own surgery. This is appreciated.

There is no doubt that for many years, and certainly at the present time, patients with chronic continuing illness of the type listed above have not received that formal, careful, follow-up and assessment that does lead ultimately to better prognosis. In simplistic terms, diabetics can be prevented from going blind and hypertensives from having strokes by the sort of formalized care described above. Increasingly, well-informed patients know this and are looking for this style of management of their conditions.

REFERENCES

1. Pendleton, D., Schofield, T., Tare, P., and Havelock, P. (1984). *The consultation: an approach to learning and teaching.* Oxford University Press.
2. Stott, N. C. H. and Davis, R. H. (1987). The exceptional potential in each primary care consultation. *In* Heller T., Bailey L., and Gott M. (eds.) *Coronary heart disease: reducing the risks. A reader.* Wiley, Chichester.
3. Office of Health Economics (1991). *Factors influencing clinical decisions in general practice.*
4. Cartwright, A. (1967). *Patients and their doctors.* Atherton Press, New York.
5. Brown, C. and Rees, W. D. W. (1990). Dyspepsia in general practice: try empirical treatment first and investigate patients who do not respond. *British Medical Journal*, **300**, 829–30.
6. Dowie, R. (1983). *General practitioners and consultants: a study of outpatient referrals.* King Edward's Hospital Fund for London, London.
7. Wilkin, D. and Smith, A. G. (1987). Variation in general practitioners' referral rates to consultants. *Journal of the Royal College of General Practitioners*, *37*, 350–3.
8. Marsh, G. N. (1982). Are follow-up consultations at medical outpatient departments futile? *British Medical Journal*, *284*, 1176–7.
9. Markus, A. C. (1986). Thyroid care. *Update*, *32*, 905–11.
10. Golding, J. (1987). Is vitamin B 12 used perniciously? *Mims Magazine*, 45–6 (1 January).
11. Shorvon, S. D., Chadwick, D., Galbraith, A. W., and Reynolds E. H. (1978). One drug for epilepsy. *British Medical Journal*, **1**, 474–6.
12. Shorvon, S. D., and Reynolds, E. H. (1979). Reduction in polypharmacy for epilepsy. *British Medical Journal*, **2**, 1023–5.
13. Sheppard, J. (1988). How one practice benefits from a nurse-run asthma clinic. *Modern Medicine*, *33*, 589–94.
14. Pearson, R. (1988). *Asthma care in general practice.* Asthma Society Training Centre, Stratford-upon-Avon.
15. Thorn, P. A. and Russell, R. G. (1973). Diabetic clinics today and tomorrow: mini-clinics in general practice. *British Medical Journal*, **2**, 534–6.
16. Mellor, J. G., Samanta, A., Blanford, R. L. *et al.* (1985). Questionnaire survey of diabetic care in general practice in Leicestershire. *Health Trends*, **17**, 61–3.

17. Waine, C. (ed.) (1988). *Diabetes*. Information folder. RCGP, London.
18. MacKinnon, M., Wilson, R. M., Hardisty, C. A. *et al.* (1989). Novel role for specialist nurses in managing diabetes in the community. *British Medical Journal*, **299**, 552–4.
19. Rohan, T. E., Frost, C. D., and Wald, N. T. (1989). Prevention of blindness by screening for diabetic retinopathy: a quantitative assessment. *British Medical Journal*, **299**, 1198–201.
20. Hart, J. T. (1987). *Hypertension: community control of high blood pressure*, 2nd edn. Churchill Livingstone, Edinburgh and London.
21. Colling, A. (1974). Home or hospital care after myocardial infarction: Is this the right question? *British Medical Journal*, **1**, 559–63.
22. McIntosh, I. B. (1987). Managing strokes at home. *Horizons*, **2**, 708–16.
23. Liddell, R., Grant, J., and Rawles J. (1990). The management of suspected myocardial infarction by Scottish general practitioners with access to community hospital beds. *British Journal of General Practice*, **40**, 318–22.
24. Pell, A. C. H., Stuart, P. C., Stewart, M. J., and Fraser D. M. (1990). Home or hospital care for acute myocardial infarction? A survey of general practitioners' attitudes in the thrombolytic era. *British Journal of General Practice*, **40**, 323–5.
25. O'Dowd, T. C., and West, R. R. (1987). Clinical prediction of Garderella vaginalis in general practice. *Journal of the Royal College of General Practitioners*, **37**, 59–61.
26. O'Dowd, T. C. (1990). New light on vaginitis. *Update*, **40**, 388–92.
27. Marsh, G. N. (1990). Auditing quality in general practice. George Swift memorial lecture. *Wessex Faculty Newsletter*.
28. Singh, B. M., Holland M. R., and Thorn P. A. (1984). Metabolic control of diabetes in general practice clinics: comparison with a hospital clinic. *British Medical Journal*, **289**, 726–8.

5. Non-prescribing and the prevention of iatrogenic disease

NON-PRESCRIBING: 'THE NULLICOPOEIA'

'In the totality of the doctor-patient interaction', as the jargon would put it—or as you and I would say, 'looking at the consultation as a whole'— the listening, the questioning, the examination, the diagnosis, the prognosis, the reassurance, and the suggestions for self-care are all important components. The medication less so. We forget this. If we remembered it, we would not be prescribing so much medication. The large amounts of poured-away drugs, the prescriptions found in litter bins, and the 'left-over' tablets at the back of medicine chests are all evidence that doctors over-prescribe for their patients.[1,2] The huge volume of self-limiting upper-respiratory-tract infections, plus the minor trauma, the transitory gastro-intestinal upsets, and the non-specific, non-serious aches and pains that form a significant proportion of general practitioners' work, do not in fact need medication.[3] They need listening, questioning, examination, explanation, collusion and reassurance. Between 1970 and 1981/2 there was a 12 per cent increase in attendance-rates for trivial complaints.[4] This was particularly evident in children in the lower social classes.

From the point of view of efficient care, an all-important factor is that minor illnesses recur. My thirty years in practice, combined with efficient continuing records, have highlighted to me how the same people do get the same illnesses and syndromes repeatedly: the same upper-respiratory-tract infections, traumas, non-specific aches and pains, gastro-intestinal upsets, depression, and so on (see Chapter 10). There is no doubt that if doctors assumed their classical role as teachers (*docere*: to teach) and educated patients in a positive way about how to manage their illnesses and their subsequent recurrences, then many many patients would not need to re-consult. Patients can certainly be taught how to assess minor illnesses themselves, and to tolerate and manage them without consultation. The place of common-sense home remedies, particularly the drinking of comforting or nourishing fluids, dietary modifications (starvation for diarrhoea), and the value of steam inhalations and simple analgesics in the ubiquitous upper-respiratory-tract infections can all be emphasized. There are now excellent leaflets available for patients with titles such as *Minor Illness—how to treat it at home*.[5] Supplies of these should be available in surgery waiting-rooms, at the reception desk (particularly during influenza epidemics), and handed out by all the clinical members of the team when they feel it appropriate. I always have a pile on my desk—obviously I am forgetting to give them out! Particularly important are the 'urgent' patients 'fitted in' that day into fully booked appointment systems; frequently they have another upper-respiratory-tract infection that they 'wish to nip in the bud', or words to that effect. Education on the limited therapy for these conditions—'there's no magic wand for this'—is vital in order to prevent similar requests in the future. At the time it can seem tempting to dash off a quick prescription, usually for ineffective antibiotics, but a little more time on education will in the long run be a more cost-effective method of dealing with these problems. This surely is a major way of preventing patients bringing every case of 'flu, sore throat, chesty cold, and diarrhoea to their doctor. If doctors medicate, to some extent it obliges patients to come for 'treatment', whereas if doctors merely advise and educate, repeat-consultations lessen. Particularly germane here is the avoidance of the prescription of antibiotics for viral respiratory infections.[6] Once patients are used to receiving antibiotics, and especially once their catarrhal children between the ages of 3½ and 7½ are medicated in this way, they come again and again. Too early exhibition of antibiotics merely results in any secondary bacterial infection being resistant to that antibiotic and requiring a second one. All those children—and I certainly have them in my practice—who seem to need all sorts of antibiotics for every upper-respiratory-tract infection and sore throat before their cure is effected are cases in point.

Some patients, or perhaps more particularly the anxious parents looking after them, observing a doctor using torch, tongue-depressor, auriscope, and stethoscope to achieve a diagnosis of self-limiting upper-respiratory-tract infection, may feel obliged to come for that alone. Hence no reduction in the consultation-rate. The prefacing of such examinations by 'from what you tell me I'll find nothing' or 'this sounds like a paracetamol-and-fluids illness' can be one way of minimizing the importance of the physical examination. Telephone consultations for repeat episodes can be easier where patients have been health-educated in the above way; a short conversation allowing them to reiterate the familiar symptoms, followed by the doctor's advice identical to the last episode—available from efficient records in front of him—is all that may be necessary. A recent influenza epidemic in the practice was largely handled on the telephone by known doctors, with records in front of them, talking to known patients (see Chapter 13).

It is important that a philosophy of self-care of minor illnesses is discussed at team meetings so that all members can help to formulate it and ultimately implement it.[3] At discussions in our own team meeting it became apparent that, apart from simple analgesics, the team members did not take minor medications themselves and neither did their families. The major reason for this appeared to be a greater awareness of the self-limiting and harmless characteristics of such illness and a more precise knowledge of the natural history. 'Tincture of time' was all-important and all that was needed.

So, if the doctor does not prescribe, this is particularly helpful to other members of the team and especially nurse, health-visitor, and midwife. They themselves cannot write prescriptions but are fully aware of the self-care management that the doctors recommend. Having protocols on the management of minor illness without the aid of medications is a useful exercise in any practice implementing a team approach.

Not only does prescribed medication reinforce in the patients' minds that consultation is necessary, but the medication itself can create extra work. Medicines cause side-effects, and if these are at all significant, such as glossitis, diarrhoea, or vaginitis, all commonly the result of antibiotics, further consultations are necessary and possibly yet more medication. Similarly, medicines produce allergic reactions—skin rashes in particular—requiring further consultation and further medication.

It is particularly important for doctors not to medicate for minor psychiatric states. Depression and anxiety are two of the commonest diagnoses in general practice.[7,8,9] These conditions could be more accurately described as 'unhappiness' and 'worry' in many patients. Uncovering the cause of their 'dis-ease'—a fairly rapid affair for a well-known doctor consulting a well-known patient—is treatment in itself.[10] I have tried not to prescribe for short-lived conditions of this type, particularly in acute crises. Drugs inhibit the motiviation for working through the problem, and sometimes make matters worse. The most important treatment seems to be that the doctor is available, known, and interested and that he listens, advises, counsels, reassures, and supports before resorting to psychotropic drugs. These measures should not be demeaned—they are what the patient has come for. Time off work is a potent treatment and is frequently all that is necessary. Drugs are not required. They should only be used when psychotherapeutic methods have failed following several consultations. Furthermore, reference to a counselling member of the team (the health-visitor for mothers with puerperal depression, a counsellor for people with interpersonal problems) can relieve the doctor of a large proportion of the continuing care, but most importantly provide more expert help than he can offer himself, and without medicating.

The continuing work-load engendered by patients addicted to psychotropics, not to mention those addicted to ineffective doctor consultations, is considerable. It often takes many hours of consultations before they can stop their drugs. Drug-and-alcohol abuse counsellors are inordinately helpful but how much better if these patients had not been prescribed habituating medication in the first place. General practitioners working in the 1970s who were inundated by drug firms producing one psychotropic panacea after another are now reaping the rewards of reliance on such medications. Conditions such as marital breakdown, anxiety state, worry, unhappiness, stress, ineffectiveness, low self-esteem, bereavement, and post-natal depression, as well as psychiatric reactions to organic disease, were all suggested targets for medicating with psychotropics. To some extent this therapeutic propaganda continues. For many of those habit-uated, the need for continuing consultations has been determined ulti-mately by the monitoring of the drug and the problem of its withdrawal, rather than the condition itself. To some extent, efficient care is synony-mous with non-medicated care.

'MINICOPOEIA'

Many general practitioners, and I am certainly one of them, spend quite a large amount of time trying to grapple with the complexities of very many different drugs. Increasingly, however, practices are trying to circumscribe the number of drugs they use and develop a 'minicopoeia'.[11,12] With a list of thirty-six reputable, rigorously tested, and commonly used drugs—all generically named—it is possible to treat over 80 per cent of the conditions seen in general practice.[13] In one minicopoeia as an example, the drugs for the cardiovascular system are limited to five—Trinitrini, Propranolol, Bendrofluazide, Digoxin, and Frusemide. By sticking to these drugs in the minicopoeia and certainly using them first in all new patients, prescribing is simplified, memory is less taxed, and because there are so few, doctors are extremely familiar with them. From continued usage they become familiar with the range of dose, likewise their interactions with other drugs. And the patients themselves will have informed their doctor of the side-effects. Other drugs and newer panaceas are prescribed only when the minicopoeia drugs fail. On the whole drugs in the minicopoeia can be cheap, and being generically named the least-expensive preparation is always dispensed. Imipramine seems to control most cases of depression and Penicillin V usually seems to work in upper-respiratory-tract infections in the over-5s requiring an antibiotic. 'Minicopocias' can be very personal but nevertheless save a great deal of time and mental effort, not to mention the other advantages.

NON-PRESCRIBING AND THE PREVENTION OF IATROGENIC DISEASE FROM THE PATIENT'S POINT OF VIEW

On the whole, patients do not like taking pills and medicine, and do not trust 'drugs'. If they can manage without them the majority of them are well pleased. They do not like the side-effects of drugs, nor do they relish iatrogenic disease. If the patients trust the doctor and feel that he understands their problem by listening and by appropriate examination, then they will accept being given no prescription and not think that the doctor is just saving money on his indicative drug budget.

I must, however, enter one caveat. In this area of non-prescribing, special care must be taken of deprived, low-social-class patients. They too can respond to health education—I have a tremendous regard for the innate intelligence of the British patient, regardless of their educational level. Nevertheless, the data does show that the socially deprived do attend more for minor illness, and this is probably associated with their low self-esteem and poor education.[4] In addition, they seek prescriptions for simple analgesics which are free of charge to them, and whose purchase would be at the expense of other vital parts of their household budget, even food, rent, and clothes. I willingly prescribe large amounts of paracetamol, for example, to such families, telling them that they are not just for the present episode but for those in the future too.

REFERENCES

1. Dunnell, K. and Cartwright, A. (1972). *Medicine takers, prescribers and hoarders*. Routledge and Kegan Paul, London.
2. Cartwright, A, and Smith, C. (1988). *Elderly people, their medicines and their doctors*. Routledge, London.
3. Marsh, G. N. (1977). 'Curing' minor illness in general practice. *British Medical Journal*, **2**, 1267–9.
4. McCormick, A., Rosenbaum, M. and Fleming, D. (1990). Socio-economic characteristics of people who consult their general practitioner. *Population Trends*, **59**, 8–10.
5. Health Education Board. *Minor Illness—and how to treat it at home*. HEB, London.
6. Stott, N. C. H. (1979). Management and outcome of winter URTIs in children, aged 0–9 years. *British Medical Journal*, **1**, 29–31.
7. Shepherd, M., Cooper, B., Brown, A. C., and Kalton, G. (1981). *Psychiatric illness in general practice*, 2nd edn. Oxford University Press.
8. Freeling, P., Downey, L. J., and Malkin, J. C. (1987). *The presentation of depression: current approaches*. Occasional Paper 36. RCGP, London.
9. Wilkinson, G. (1989). *Depression: recognition and treatment in general practice*. Radcliffe, Oxford.
10. Balin, M. (1957). *The doctor, his patient and the illness*. Pitman, London.
11. Grant, G. B., Gregory, D. A., and Zwanenberg, T. D. van (1987). *A basic formulary for general practice*. Oxford University Press.
12. Royal College of General Practitioners Northern Ireland Faculty (1988). *Practice formulary, 1988–1990*, RCGP, London.
13. Marsh, G. N. (1981). Stringent prescribing in general practice. *British Medical Journal*, **283**, 1159–60.

6. Repeat prescribing

By repeat prescribing is meant the giving of a prescription where there is no doctor-patient consultation immediately around its time of issue. Despite the fact that this type of medicating has received much criticism, this chapter will argue that repeat prescriptions can render the care of clinical conditions extremely efficient, markedly reduce the need for consultations, and carry benefit rather than detriment to individual patients.[1,2,3] That patients so understand their illness that they can be permitted to order their own medication and alter it appropriately, I consider to be the ultimate in good health education. Patently there have to be safeguards, and these will be discussed.[4]

There are three broad types of illness which lend themselves to the issuing of repeat prescriptions and examples of these are listed in Table 6.1. Some of the illnesses could be under more than two headings, but detail is unimportant for the purposes of discussing repeat prescriptions.

ILLNESSES REQUIRING LONG-TERM OR PERMANENT THERAPY

Establishment of the diagnosis of illnesses of this type frequently necessitates several consultations including some with other members of the primary health-care team. Let me illustrate with one or two examples.

Hypertension

Repetitive estimation of blood-pressure and appropriate tests (blood, urine, ECG, and so on) by the practice nurse is necessary to diagnose hypertension. However, once this important diagnosis has been established accurately and the appropriate medication found, the intervals between consultations can increase considerably. Patients can be left to obtain repeat prescriptions without further doctor consultation and occasionally attend the vascular clinic to see the nurse (see Chapter 4). Any change in the patient's blood-pressure will be discussed with the appropriate doctor and the repeat prescription modified.

Acne vulgaris

Teenage acne is not a difficult diagnosis, although two or three supportive and sympathetic early consultations are well received whilst treatments

Table 6.1   *Illnesses lending themselves to repeat prescriptions*

Illnesses requiring long-term or permanent therapy
Hypertension*
Acne*
Epilepsy
Angina
Congestive heart failure
Thyroid deficiency

Illnesses which remit and exacerbate
Bronchial asthma*
Hay fever*
Sinusitis*
Eczema
Otitis externa

Isolated episodes of illness which repeat themselves from time to time
Vaginal discharge*
Backache and sciatica*
Cervical spondylosis*
Migraine
Acute cystitis

---

* Discussed in text.

are assessed. Thereafter the taking of, for example, Oxytetracycline (or other similar preparation), accompanied by detergent at night, and possibly the use of a cream containing a keratolytic agent may well control a condition that can last for several years. Patients can be advised to reduce the medication from twice to once daily if suppression has proved effective. An information leaflet can substantiate the doctor's advice as well as increase the patient's knowledge of her illness.

ILLNESSES WHICH REMIT AND EXACERBATE

Bronchial asthma

Asthma is well known to run a chronic yet eminently controllable course. It exacerbates when extrinsic factors worsen—upper-respiratory-tract infection, exposure to dust or pollen, exercise, and so on—and it is the education of individual patients as to what to do in such circumstances that is the essence of self-management. For example, asthmatics who exacerbate in response to virus infections must be taught to increase their inhaled selective beta 2-adrenoceptor stimulants (for example, Salbutamol) immediately, rendering airways open and drainage of mucus effective. They must also be taught that antibiotics are not indicated, unless their temperature rises persistently and is associated with purulent sputum and lack of response to inhalations. Asthmatics can also be advised when to introduce steroid inhalants, how to vary the dose, and the duration of their use. For the few asthmatics who need oral steroids, they too can be taught to titrate their dosage against their bronchospasm. Severe asthmatics should always have steroid tablets available. They must also know the indications for further consultation. Self-assessment using prescribed peak-flow meters is now commonplace and is another aid to self-care. The ready availability of repeat prescriptions for a minimum of two inhalers of each type each time, and oral preparations given out in large amounts, should prevent the disaster of 'running out'. However, receptionists must be made aware that if asthma inhalers are requested urgently on a Saturday morning this should be looked upon as an emergency and a repeat prescription organized immediately.

Hay fever

Patients with hay fever should not need to consult each year. After some 'experience' they will know well enough what regime is best for them and can request and receive appropriate repeat prescriptions. The educational advice given by the doctor—the closed night window, the pollen-free bedroom, the avoidance of dust and minimizing exposure to certain flowers and grasses—will patently reduce symptoms, but most patients with hay fever will require tablets and/or topical nasal and ocular preparations. They should be readily available on request.

Sinusitis

Many people get recurrent episodes of maxillary or frontal sinusitis. It is usually triggered by an upper-respiratory-tract infection and they are well aware of it developing and know the importance of steam inhalations as an attempt to prevent it. Nevertheless, antibiotics are often required and repeat prescriptions for these would not seem inappropriate.

EPISODES OF ILLNESS WHICH REPEAT THEMSELVES FROM TIME TO TIME

It seems from my lifetime experience of caring for the same group of patients over many years that people do seem to get the same illnesses recurrently. (I am sorry to keep repeating this but its realization is extremely important.) This is true not only of continuing illnesses such as asthma but also relatively minor illnesses. Patients are only too well-aware of their symptoms and, if suitably health-educated in previous episodes, will also be aware of the appropriate medication. All they need is a prompt repeat prescription. For such patients (and their doctor) the consultation is an unnecessary elaboration.

Vaginal discharge

Many women get repeated episodes of vaginal discharge, particularly in their sexually active and child-bearing years. They become quite expert at diagnosing them, particularly the ubiquitous monilia whose thick, white, irritating discharge is so characteristic. They are also well aware of precipitating factors, such as taking broad-spectrum antibiotics. Hence repeat prescriptions for courses of Clotrimazole in a form previously found effective seem logical. Such patients are sufficiently well informed to know that if the therapy is unsuccessful they can attend the practice nurse for further assessment, possibly including high-vaginal swab. It is well known that some women use natural yogurt to treat their vaginal discharges very satisfactorily, and the leaving of prescriptions merely furthers this principle.

Backache, sciatica, and neck-ache

Lumbago and sciatica, and also neck-ache and brachial neuralgia, come and go in those susceptible. Repeat prescriptions for previously effective non-steroidal anti-inflammatory preparations, coupled with their know-ledge of other appropriate therapy—initially rest, heat, possibly corset or collar, then gradual mobility and exercises—are all that is required. The patients' previous knowledge, this time of pain, very rapidly tells them whether the course or severity is different and whether they need to consult.

CONTROLS ON REPEAT PRESCRIBING

'Rubbish'

It should go without saying, although probably in every practice, and certainly in mine, it does not, that ineffective remedies—'rubbish'—should not find their way into the repeat-prescribing system. Hence computers should not generate repeat prescriptions for expectorants, linctuses, counter-irritants, and anti-diarrhoeal preparations, to name but a few. Hopefully patients with coughs, colds, sore throats, aches and pains, diarrhoeas, and so on—the multiplicity of minor illnesses for which only time is needed—will have been educated by all members of the team as to how to manage these illnesses without recourse to medication, or perhaps by seeking simple symptom-relief from the local chemist (see Chapter 5). One advantage of having many repeat prescriptions on computer is that from time to time the list can be scrutinized and the presence of ineffective remedies questioned.

Availability

No matter which system is used—repeat-prescription cards, computerized slips, and so on—it is virtually impossible to provide all repeat prescriptions immediately on demand. However, for some patients who take their tablets with extreme regularity—women taking the contraceptive pill are a good example—the computer can be programmed to issue the repeats prior to their arrival at the surgery. If they are then to see the family-planning nurse for a check-up at that time, she can hand out those already signed prescriptions. But for many patients their repeats seem to be so erratic, or their medication so complex, that when requests are made a twenty-four-hour delay in receiving the prescription is unavoidable.

Number of repeats

There must be a limit to the number of prescriptions that can be issued before records are scrutinized or the patient is told to reconsult. In my own practice, the majority of repeat medications have a 'stop' put on them usually after one year, or sometimes after eighteen months, has passed from the ordaining of the repeat prescription. This does not necessarily mean that further consultation must take place, but it does mean that the doctor is made aware of the repeat prescriptions that are being issued and can look at the patient's records. Obviously, reconsultation will depend on what particular drug is involved and the condition for which it is being used. For some drugs, however, a quicker 'stop' is put on the prescription, and this particularly applies to psychotropic drugs where the interval is usually every three months. It should be remembered incidentally that when the 'stop' on a repeat prescription operates it is not necessarily with the doctor that the patient reconsults. For example, it may be more appropriate for a controlled schizophrenic to see the community psychiatric nurse or a hypertensive the practice nurse.

Amounts prescribed

The volume of drugs needs to be considered carefully but not necessarily too stringently. In my own practice many patients taking one or two tablets daily will receive six months' supply, and others taking three or four tablets per day an eighty-four-day supply. There can be great flexibility according to the drug, the condition, and the individual patient. Repeat prescriptions are very much a 'tailor-made' operation. As an illustrative example, there seems no reason why a patient with long-controlled thyroid deficiency should not receive 365 tablets of appropriate strength Thyroxine.

Hospital 'repeats'

Many patients, particularly the elderly, begin continuing medication on discharge from hospital. It is important to scrutinize this carefully, first to ensure that the generic name is being used, and secondly, that the particular preparation is in the practice 'minicopoeia'—if it is not, and the practice 'minicopoeia' contains a virtually identical alternative then the patient can be switched to that (see Chapter 5). Thirdly, general practitioners should not be afraid to stop medication which they feel may have been appropriate in hospital but is no longer necessary now that the patient is at home.

THE VOLUME OF REPEAT PRESCRIPTIONS

It is estimated that half of all prescriptions are written without a consultation taking place.[5] Prior to computers this involved reception staff in a large amount of record-checking and prescription-writing. It is of interest that the earliest computer programmes to be used in general practice were the ones for repeat prescriptions. Those who criticize this system of care should weigh in their minds this pragmatic response of busy general practitioners to their patients' illnesses. My personal philosophy of patients taking a greater responsibility for the care of their illnesses would in fact increase the proportion of prescriptions written without a consultation.

Views vary as to which particular drugs are being given most on repeat prescriptions, but the consensus seems to be that drugs for the control of hypertension and for respiratory infections are commonest, and that psychotropics, which were very common, are now becoming less so. In my own practice, the computer shows that the two commonest drugs issued on repeat prescription were Salbutamol inhalers for asthmatics, followed by Co-Proxamol for the various chronic pains to which many patients are subject. They were followed by Cimetidine and/or Ranitidine for hyperacidic disorders of the oesophagus, stomach, and duodenum. Following this came Ibuprofen for numerous musculo-skeletal pains, varying in severity from the rheumatoid and osteo-arthritics to the non-specific musculo-skeletal aches and pains that are endemic in the community. Thyroxine for the thyroid-deficient came next, followed by five drugs all used for the treatment of various forms of cardio-vascular disease: Glyceryl trinitrate,

Bendrofluazide, Atenolol, Frusemide, and Digoxin. Those are my practice's 'top ten' and all in my 'minicopoeia' (see Chapter 5).

Some critics of repeat prescribing seem to imply that patients almost universally wish to cheat, exploit or otherwise abuse the system. In my experience, the vast majority of patients are responsible citizens who, once they are well-informed on their illness, are only too keen to take a cautious approach to its medication. Nevertheless, a reliable repeat-prescription card system is desirable, and Figure 6.1 shows the repeat prescription which was used in my practice for many years. The patients merely indicated on a slip of paper alongside the letter of the particular drug they required, and left the card at the reception desk or in a box in the waiting-room. The prescription was waiting twenty-four hours later. Now the computer itself generates a list of the drugs that the patient is on (Figure 6.2), and indicates to the patient how often they can be repeated before a check is necessary.

The ultimate aim should be immediate provision of repeat prescriptions: the patient arrives at reception window and leaves with signed prescription a few minutes later. But as I said earlier, with the doctor's signature essential and doctors occupied in other ways, this is virtually impossible. In addition, the computer may be in use for other 'functions' and not be able to generate a prescription at a moment's notice. Nevertheless, for acute episodes, for example, 'another sticky eye', 'a recurrence of cystitis' (this on a Saturday morning), an immediate repeat prescription is essential and allowances should be made for this (see also the earlier paragraph on urgent availability of asthma therapy). For prescriptions for continuing or recurrent illness, however, a twenty-four-hour delay between request and provision seems reasonable. Many patients send requests by post with stamped, addressed envelope enclosed. The elderly know that when bottles of medication are perhaps two-thirds empty the time has come to order their repeat.

From time to time, and with the best organization in the world, some patients—particularly those less cerebrally endowed—will come for consultation for 'just a repeat of my tablets doctor'. This is an opportunity, not for repeating the prescription, but for education about future behaviour. They can be made aware (probably not for the first time) that staff are employed for this purpose, either for the checking and writing the prescriptions, or for using the computer, and that such consultations with the doctor are inappropriate. All this is spelled out in the nicest possible way.

Receptionists faced with requests for repeat prescriptions from patients for whom there is no evidence, either in the records or on the computer, that one has been ordained can check with the appropriate doctor to see whether the request is reasonable and whether it should become a permanent repeat arrangement. Usually the answer is yes. Hence, little by little, more and more patients have the facility to request repeat prescriptions.

●

KEEP CAREFULLY

To obtain a repeat prescription without seeing the Doctor, leave this card at the surgery in an unsealed, self-addressed envelope and collect your prescription on the following day, after 11.30 a.m.

If you stamp your envelope it will be posted to you.

Please let us know the letters or name of which items you require. The name of your tablet, medicine, etc. will be shown on the chemist's label.

N.B. In order to eliminate errors, we can no longer accept orders for prescriptions by telephone.

●

Dr. G.N. MARSH

Dr. R. G. P. HALL

Dr. J. R. THORNHAM

Dr. R. A. HORNE

Dr. D. H. WHITE

DR. F. E. GRIFFITHS   DR. C. P. O'NEILL

NORTON MEDICAL CENTRE,
HARLAND HOUSE
NORTON,
STOCKTON-ON-TEES,
CLEVELAND.

Telephone: Stockton 360111 (4 lines)

Please notify loss of this card immediately.

PLEASE BRING THIS CARD WITH YOU WHEN YOU COME TO SEE THE DOCTOR

Surname, Mr., Mrs., Miss ....

Christian Names ....

Address ....

DESCRIPTION OF MEDICINE :

A Tab. Atenolon 100mg ....
   1 daily   200
   ....

B Beconase   2 ....
   2 puffs bd
   ....

C Tab Chlorpheniramine 4mg ....
   1 tds   150
   ....

D ....
   ....

E ....
   ....

F ....
   ....

Date of renewal	Items
14.5.89	A, B, C
30.6.89	C
18.8.89	B, C
1.10.89	C
12.11.89	A, B, C

Fig. 6.1.   Repeat-prescription card

COST

With the indicative drug budgets, it is important to consider whether the cost of repeat prescribing will be higher than if consultations always

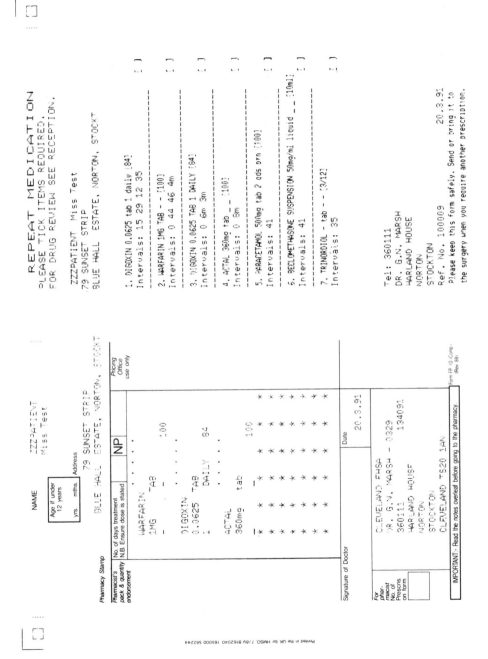

Fig. 6.2.   Computerized repeat medication

ensued. There is no hard and fast data on this, only surmise. It is my belief that patients receiving large amounts of medication, who are well informed and health-educated—and I repeat how bright the socially deprived or other formally ill-educated British patients are—will use the repeat-prescription system carefully. Remember also that if patients receive twelve months' supply of Thyroxine tablets, they will also reduce the work of the receptionist and the computer. As a result of the small number of prescriptions written (that is, large amounts are given on each one), the dispensing fees will be considerably reduced. They are not an inconsiderable amount in the total NHS drug bill. By the same token, in that the repeat prescriptions are all for items that are generic, that are for the most part the cheapest available, and that exclude any ineffective remedies, the cost-effectiveness of therapy will be high. All in all, therefore, I do not believe that a practice with a large number of repeat prescriptions, ordained along the lines spelled out, will produce a high drug bill. My own is about two-thirds of the national average in an area noted for its high morbidity.

REPEAT PRESCRIBING FROM THE PATIENT'S POINT OF VIEW

An efficient, generous, repeat-prescribing system has many benefits to patients. Firstly, it gives them ready access to their medicines when they need them. Secondly, as part of the education preceding a repeat prescription, they will of necessity learn more about their clinical condition. They will learn about their illness's self-care, prior to the need for medication, and also learn when it is appropriate to re-consult. These are all areas which patients describe as being difficult when asked about the problems of seeing their doctor. The busy patient is freed from having to consult. Many patients obliged to re-consult merely for a repeat prescription feel guilty about 'wasting the doctor's time'. But above all it puts *their* illness in *their* hands; to me, and I hope an increasing number of doctors, this seems eminently appropriate. It is important that the doctor avoids making patients feel that he does not want to see them. The message to be got across by the entire team—and perhaps especially by the receptionists—is that the appointments system is always open, but if patients do not feel the need to consult then repeat prescribing is available.

REFERENCES

1. Balint, M., Hurst, J., Joyce, D., Marinker, M., and Woodcock, J. (1970 first published, 1984 reprint). *Treatment or diagnosis: a study of repeat prescriptions in general practice*. Tavistock, London.

2. Nicol, F. and Gebbie, H. (1984) Repeat prescribing in the elderly. A case for audit? *Scottish Medical Journal*, **29**, 21–24.
3. Difford, F. (1984). Reducing prescribing costs through computer controlled repeat prescribing. *Journal of the Royal College of General Practitioners*, **34**, 658–60.
4. Steel, K., Mills, A., Gilliland, A. E. W. *et al.* (1987). Repeat prescribing of non-steroidal anti-inflammatory drugs excluding aspirin: how careful are we? *British Medical Journal*, **295**, 962–4.
5. Mapes, R. (ed.) (1980). *Prescribing practice and drug usage*. Croom Helm, London.

7. Preventative care

GENERAL PRINCIPLES

It goes without saying that if all illness were preventable this would be an extremely efficient method of care. Hence this chapter is the longest one in the book. To give two examples, if all children were immunized against measles then the work involved in caring for the current epidemics would disappear. By the same token, screening of all patients for hypertension, particularly males between 40 and 65, could prevent the enormous volume of work associated with a 'young stroke'.[1,2] So, as you get embroiled in the, perhaps, tedious detail of preventative protocols and so on later in this chapter, remember that prevention is an efficient method of care. Remember too that the vast majority of preventative care is actually undertaken by the non-doctor members of the team. Hence the doctor has more time to use his diagnostic skills on undifferentiated problems, as well as the planning of management of illness, which are components of the team's care probably unique to him. Perhaps it should be stressed at this time, without appearing sexist, that female doctors are particularly at risk of being drawn into the preventative-care field. Areas such as family planning, paediatric surveillance, antenatal care, and well-woman checks have been almost traditionally associated with female doctors;[3] they can mostly be done by nurses, midwives, health-visitors, and so on.

Preventative care itself has to be efficient. The volume of it is huge if all children are to have comprehensive paedriatric surveillance, if all well adults are to be checked every three or five years, if the elderly are to be seen every year, and if family planning, antenatal care, and so on are to be done appropriately for everyone. So it is important for doctors, who may well be responsible for co-ordinating the policies involved in preventative care, to have cognizance of the volume problem and the need for an efficient cost-effective programme for the team members actually doing the work. This more particularly since it is well known that there is a hard core of people—frequently of low social class and also deprived—who do not present themselves or their children for their preventative care, yet have a greater need for it.[4] Cost-effective care releases time for such people.

TEAM MEMBERS AND QUALIFICATIONS

Doctors

So, having dismissed the doctor as almost irrelevant to the majority of preventative care in a team setting, what remains for him to do? It is he who is overall most responsible for the care being carried out and co-ordinated for the patients registered with him. In addition, there are some 'bits' in the preventative-care protocols that only he can do. For example, he has to do the physical examination of a new-born and six-week-old baby, although the majority of the paediatric programme is undertaken by the health-visitor (Table 7.1). There is no doubt that the doctor receives training in preventative care at his medical school, and much knowledge. Nevertheless, other members of the team have similar and perhaps more intense training, particularly health-visitors, and perhaps most importantly look upon it as mainstream to their work. As a result they continue to keep up to date, primarily by doing the work as a principal task, but also by attending courses, lectures, and other continuing forms of postgraduate instruction. So the doctor becomes out of date whilst the other preventative-health-care workers continue to develop and update their knowledge. Obviously all health-care workers, including the doctors, will do some opportunistic preventative care in their normal consultations: for example, they will (or should) remember to mention the dangers of smoking when talking to adult patients or the importance of sound contraception when dealing with the sexually active. But, apart from this kind of care, aided particularly by preventative-care sheets in the record or on a computer screen, the doctor's main role in prevention is taking responsibility for its being done: for seeing that the programmes are cost-effective and that they are facilitated and carried out by other more skilled and informed members of the primary health-care team.

Health-visitors

The main role of the health-visitor is a preventative one. Qualified as a registered general nurse, with some midwifery training, followed by a twelve-month course orientated on preventative care at a college of education, she is established as a major worker in prevention in the primary health-care team. Traditionally, she has worked with children and expectant mothers, but in some areas of Great Britain she has widened her preventative remit to other groups, increasingly the elderly. This enormous work-load relieves doctors of a large amount of care. Her involvement with patients antenatally, co-ordinating that care with the midwives who are the main carers at that time, coupled with her statutory

Table 7.1   *Pre-school paediatric surveillance protocol*

Done by	Age of child	Parameters checked
Paediatrician or general practitioner	Birth (within 24 hours)	Review family history, parental concerns. Weight, head circumference. Full physical examination—in particular: inspect eyes, red reflexes, heart-sounds, hips, genitalia, testes.
Paediatrician or general practitioner	5–10 days	Review parents' concerns. Check eyes, hips. Full physical examination in absence of recorded birth examination available to GP. PKU, thyroid function.
General practitioner or clinical medical officer	6 weeks (coincides with mother's post-natal examination)	General parental concerns, particuarly re. vision and hearing. Weight, head circumference. Physical examination—particularly eyes, red reflexes, heart-sounds, hips, testes, head control, tone, etc.
Health-visitor	7–9 months	General parental concerns, particularly vision and hearing. Weight, testes, hips (*not* Barlow/Ortolani method). Look for squint, observe visual behaviour—refer on suspicion or strong family history of visual defect. Use distraction test for hearing. Be aware of significant incidence of iron deficiency anaemia in pre-school children (up to 10%)
Health-visitor	18–24 months	Parental concerns, particularly behaviour, vision, and hearing. Check speech is beginning, and understanding of speech.
Health-visitor	36–42 months	Ask about vision, squint, hearing, behaviour, development. Height (plot). Check heart sounds, testes (GP). Hearing test if indicated.

Source: Based on the Hall Report (D. M. B. Hall (ed.), *Health for all children*. Oxford; OUP).

visit to the baby after birth, establish her in the mother's eyes as someone to whom she can turn for continuing care of her baby.[5] In particular, in the antenatal period, the health-visitor should be seeing all teenage and single-parent pregnancies, socially and financially deprived mothers, grand multipara, women considering adoption of their baby, and women coping with physical illness as well as pregnancy. Her advice regarding diet, exercise, hygiene, and arrangements for the baby are all important areas. Once the baby is born, the health-visitor carries out a statutory fourteen-day visit which leads on to her main role in the entire programme of developmental paediatric care (see Chapter 7). With her expanding remit, this can lead into preventative care in adult life.

Midwife

Antenatal care is a major exercise in preventative care, and the midwife has the major role.[6] Like much preventative care, it is done according to protocol, and the details are spelled out later in this chapter. Suffice to say that the old-fashioned system of antenatal attendances—monthly to thirty-two weeks, fortnightly to thirty-six weeks, and weekly until delivery—a system ordained for the socially deprived and physically handicapped women of the 1930s, is now no longer necessary.[7] Both midwife and doctor attendances can be reduced (see later). The midwife enjoys her preventative care, and much of her training orientates around that aspect of midwifery.

Family-planning nurse

In some teams the midwife does the family planning also, but it is more common for the family-planning nurse to be a registered general nurse (with or without midwifery experience) who has attended the family-planning course recognized by the English National Board for Nursing Midwifery and Health Visiting (Course No. 900). When I attended my GP Family-Planning Course it was run jointly with nurses. The course-content was identical for both doctors and nurses, except that the former learnt how to insert intra-uterine devices and the latter studied organization of clinics, sterilization of instruments, and so on. Hence, the family-planning nurse has virtually as much knowledge of the subject as her doctor colleague, and can undertake most of the day-to-day consultative care. The family-planning nurse works to two major protocols, one for the assessment of patients starting contraception for the first time, and the second for the ongoing supervision of patients already established on contraception. In my own practice, the family-planning nurse does about 300 consultations per doctor per year—a considerable work-load previously done by the doctor until she became a member of the team.[8] Pre-conception counselling can be neatly co-ordinated with family planning, and the nurse does this also.[9] Again a protocol is necessary (see later). Finally (at least for the present) our nurse has started a menopause and HRT clinic, since much of the advice concerns the prevention of osteoporosis in some women in later life.

Community-nursing sisters

Like all registered general nurses, the community-nursing sisters have had basic training in preventative care. Furthermore, their community-nursing course contains further instructions in preventative care. Sadly, however, many of them have little time to implement this training.[10,11] Most of their time is spent in bedside nursing in the community, but they do see the elderly a great deal, and can do opportunistic preventative care. For example, they can become aware of the psycho-social limitations of an elderly person's way of life—need for easier food supplies, chiropody, handicapped aids, social contact, home-helps, and so on—and also detect hazards in the home like loose mats, awkward steps, difficult stairs, and defective electrics. Thus they can practice their preventative-care training. Given enough time, they can extend their work to checking urines of the overweight elderly for diabetes, taking blood-pressures, and giving advice about weight, diet and the like. Unfortunately the community-nursing 'hierarchy' tend to be somewhat restrictive about what community nurses can and cannot do, and are particularly discouraging with regard to them spending more time in practice premises carrying out clinic-style work. Given extra training, they could do well-person, family-planning, and vascular clinics, and undertake other duties, but their major 'official' role is seen as taking nursing into the homes of the people in the community, even though that community is fitter and more mobile, and increasingly able and prepared to travel to them. This is not meant to devalue the excellent and vital home-based care of the very frail, the house-bound handicapped, the seriously ill, the dying—merely to underline that the volume of that care is shrinking, whilst the potential for preventative care of the whole community is expanding.

Practice nurse

The practice nurse is the main preventative-care worker in many primary health-care teams.[12,13] Reference to Table 1 shows that over two-thirds of her work is preventative. In my practice, her most common consultations were for tetanus and travel immunizations (21 per cent of her preventative work), cervical smears and well-person clinics (27 per cent), and paediatric immunizations (15 per cent). She works to protocols in preventative care in much the same way as the midwife uses protocols for her antenatal care. These protocols have developed from joint discussions with the doctors in the practice. It is of paramount importance that the nurse herself is involved in formulating the protocols so that she does not undertake work outside her competence and for which she is untrained. Occasionally, the doctors have to teach nurses how to carry out procedures with which they may not be familiar (for example, taking cervical smears or ECGs). Analyses of the tasks carried out at the various preventative-care clinics indicate that her basic registered-general-nurse training, albeit mostly carried out in a hospital setting, is the core of her knowledge. This training obviously includes clinical knowledge of diseases, diagnostic techniques such as blood-pressure estimation, taking throat-swabs, injections, and dressings, as well as more behaviourally orientated expertise, including particularly the ability to relate to and communicate with patients. It is probable that two or three years in post as a staff nurse on a busy medical or surgical hospital ward is valuable preparation for the varied clinical tasks of the practice nurse.

Where care is being given to all age-groups and all social classes, life experience—courtship, marriage, motherhood—is of inordinate value. The clinically experienced nurse who is married and has brought up children is probably ideally suited to the varied preventative care that she will undertake. The one area in which our own practice nurse felt further training would be helpful was in counselling skills, and a programme was available at a local college of further education. No matter which part of her work she was doing, she has found these skills useful. Once in post, and carrying out preventative-care clinics, she can 'hand over' to further nurses coming into the practice. Such a hand-over period may well need to be as long as three months, in order that as many aspects of care as possible can be seen. The nurse must be prepared to 'read up' her expanding preventative-care role. There are an increasing number of practice-nurse courses, and these contain a large preventative content.[14,15,16]

Like the doctor in the practice, the practice nurse should be allocated one half-day per week for study. During this period she can read relevant articles, discuss problems with other members of the team, and design new, or modify old, protocols. In addition, she car visit libraries, laboratories, colposcopy clinics, district immunizatio clinics, and so on. Although there are a considerable number of ꞓrmal, comprehensive, practice-nurse-training programmes, many practice nurses were in post and functioning effectively before these existed.[17] It seems, therefore, that in the development of a primary health-care team, a reasonably well-experienced clinical nurse can gradually 'grow' into the preventative part of her job. Nevertheless, a formal training or series of courses designed around the work would appear to be desirable and prove to be of increasing value in the future, if not even mandatory.[18,19] The practice nurse will need to be flexible, not only regarding the content of her job but also as to when her services are provided. Increasingly, evening and Saturday clinics will be expected by the working population.

Elderly-care visitor

The work of the elderly-care visitor is almost entirely preventative. There are a large number of services available in most communities, such as domiciliary hairdressing, chiropody, meals on wheels, library service, and laundry facilities. Many of them are unknown to general practitioners but the elderly-care visitor, informed of them all, can discuss with elderly patients in the practice what their needs are, and facilitate appropriate provision. An elderly-care-visitor service was provided in my practice and funded by a partner's research grant in the late 1980s.[20] It was extremely popular with our elderly patients and has provided a protocol for the elderly care now mandatory under the 'new contract'.

Clinical medical officers

The clinical medical officer can liaise with the primary health-care team (see Chapter 1). He can be of considerable value in designing protocols for developmental paediatrics, immunizations, and so on, and be a link with the school medical services. It is possible that, if primary health-care teams work effectively, the work of the clinical medical officer on a day-to-day, clinic-by-clinic, basis could dwindle, and his expertise could then be more of an advisory nature. Some teams ask district clinical medical officers to undertake the preventative care and paediatric development of children in their practice, working alongside the health-visitors and according to their practice protocols.

PROTOCOLS FOR PREVENTATIVE-CARE CLINICS

Because of the constantly evolving nature of preventative care, protocols for clinics change from day to day. Accordingly, those that follow are merely examples that happen to work in my practice at the present time. Even by today's standards they are imperfect, but they do indicate a serious attempt to carry out this work in a caring and efficient way. Readers can feel free to copy them, or, more probably, use them as jumping-off points for better ones.

Pre-school surveillance

The pre-school surveillance protocol (Table 7.1) is based on the contents of the Hall Report.[21] The important thing to note is that after the early physical checks the rest of the work is done by the health-visitor. At 36–42 months the health-visitor calls in the doctor to check for maldescent of testes and absence of significant cardiac murmurs: usually a one-minute job. Suffice to say that, with the doctor and health-visitor working through this protocol in a co-ordinated way for each child, there should be no delayed recognition of physical defects (congenital dislocation of the hip, undescended testes, important cardiac murmurs), or delay in spotting slow physical, mental, or emotional development, or tardy attention to problems with the special senses.

Paediatric immunizations

Probably in most practices now, immunization of babies and children has become the work of the practice nurse. The programme is ordained by the Department of Health and varies from time to time; Table 7.2 shows the latest version. Mothers of babies and children are advised about immunization by the health-visitor at her statutory fourteen-day visit and thereafter. When the doctor carries out the mother's six-week postnatal examination and the baby's preventative-care check, he can reinforce the need for full immunization.[22] The practice nurse sets aside special times for her clinic and needs a doctor immediately available to her within the building. Her knowledge of paedriatric immunizations should be the most up-to-date of all members of the primary health-care team (including the doctor). Increasingly, practice nurses are recording the immunizations directly on to desk-top computers for central auditing and to facilitate recall. By using the above system, and particularly by checking on and chasing up defaulters—largely the work of the health-visitor—illnesses such as measles and whooping cough should be completely eliminated. Many practices have now achieved this.

Family-planning clinic

Figure 7.1 shows a typical family-planning record card, which can be readily adapted to a computer screen, and the headings more or less constitute the clinical protocol to which the practice family-planning nurse works.[8] Those considering starting contraception sometimes see their own doctor to discuss alternative methods, but many go directly to the nurse. After the nurse has taken a relevant history according to the headings on the card, she and the patient decide on the most appropriate form of contraception.

Oral contraceptives.
If the woman decides on the pill, routine blood-pressure, breast palpation, and a cervical smear are carried out. If the patient has seen only the nurse,

Table 7.2   *Immunization schedule: effective from 1 May 1990*

Vaccine	Age		Notes
Diphtheria, tetanus, pertussis, and polio	1st dose	2 months	
	2nd dose	3 months	Primary course
	3rd dose	4 months	
Measles, mumps, rubella (MMR)		12–18 months	Can be given at any age over 12 months
Booster diptheria, tetanus, and polio		4–5 years	
Measles, mumps, rubella (MMR)			If not given earlier
Rubella		10–14 years	GIRLS ONLY
BCG		10–14 years or infancy	Interval of 3 weeks between BCG and rubella
Booster tetanus and polio		15–18 years	

CHILDREN should therefore have received the following vaccines:

By 6 months:	3 doses of diphtheria, tetanus, pertussis and polio, or diphtheria, tetanus, and polio
By 18 months:	Measles, mumps, rubella
By school entry:	4th diphtheria, tetanus and polio; measles, mumps, rubella if missed earlier
Between 10 and 14 years:	BCG; rubella for girls
Before leaving school:	5th polio and tetanus

ADULTS should receive the following vaccines:

Women sero-negative for rubella:	Rubella
Previously unimmunized individuals:	Polio, tetanus.
Individuals in high-risk groups:	Hepatitis B, influenza

the doctor may wish to see the patient to examine the heart for previously undetected valve lesions and as a double-check for suitability for oral contraception.

Intra-uterine device

If an intra-uterine device is thought most appropriate, this is inserted by the doctor with the nurse assisting. The nurse checks six weeks after

FAMILY PLANNING RECORD

Christian Name:

Surname:

D.O.B.

Family History: Stroke:

Diabetes:

Other:

Gynae. Opn.:

Thrombosis:

V.V.'s:

Depressive:

Epilepsy:

Illness:

Parity:

Gravidity:

Medical History: Serious Illness:

Headache: Migraine:

Heart Disease: Jaundice:

Menstrual Formula ———

Date	Notes	Method or Name of Pill	Weight	Urine	BP	VE	Smear

Fig. 7.1. Family-planning clinic record card

Table 7.3   *Family-planning clinic protocol: run by a nurse for women established on contraception*

Yearly history
3-yearly smear
Yearly—weight
           —blood-pressure
Hb if indicated
Discuss problems with doctor

insertion that the threads are visible and that the patient has no untoward symptoms. Yearly follow-up is then carried out by the nurse.

Diaphragm
Doctor measures and nurse checks thereafter.

Continuing supervision
Regardless of the contraceptive method, the family-planning nurse carries out the continuing care according to the protocol in Table 7.3.

In pregnancy
During the last few weeks of pregnancy the midwife should routinely advise all women to see the family-planning nurse to discuss method of contraception after pregnancy. The subject is again discussed by the health-visitor at her statutory visit fourteen days after the birth and by the doctor at the six-week postnatal examination. The family-planning nurse is therefore closely linked with the health-visitor and midwife during and after pregnancy.

Home visits and follow-up
By seeing the community nurses, health-visitors, and social workers frequently at morning team meetings, the family-planning nurse can 'contact' those women in greatest need of contraceptive advice—frequently those least likely to seek it. She can pay home visits herself to deprived patients and single mothers. In my own practice she has even brought anxious mothers to the surgery for insertion of intra-uterine devices. She can also follow up problems of a preventative type, such as smoking, obesity, and hypertension, as part of her routine clinic work.

With nurse-run family-planning clinics in the surgery, the doctor's role is largely opportunistic. He can introduce the subject of contraception in consultations around teenage problems, abortion (spontaneous or induced), menstrual disturbances, marital problems, and when talking to

Table 7.4 *Protocol for pre-conception counselling*

Age	Family history
Contraception	Dating periods
Cervical smear	Rubella antibodies
Smoking	Alcohol
Diet and exercise	Weight
Diseases (e.g. diabetes, blood-pressure)	Drugs (Proprietary and prescribed)
Low social class	Ethnic minorities

newly registered patients. Appropriate people can be directed to the family-planning nurse for advice and care. The result of all these co-ordinated efforts should mean that the number of unplanned and unwanted pregnancies is small and requests for termination of pregnancy minimal. Prevention of this sort ultimately means that less overall care is needed.

Pre-conception counselling clinic

Table 7.4 shows the protocol used by an appropriately trained family-planning nurse for pre-conception counselling.[9] Most of the headings are 'common sense' for any medical or nursing member of the team. They were arrived at in the customary way by discussion between the nurse and the doctors. Of particular interest is that, despite the fact that pre-conception counselling is a relatively new concept and not found in many practices, the clinic itself is run by appropriately trained nurses working to a protocol. Innovations are not the sole prerogative of doctors.

Antenatal and postnatal care

As I suggested earlier in this chapter, the current conventional system of antenatal care—monthly to thirty-two weeks, fortnightly until thirty-six weeks, and weekly until delivery—was ordained for socially deprived and physically handicapped women of the 1930s. It is now no longer necessary. The work of Marion Hall in Aberdeen indicates clearly that this traditional system of care has proved no more effective in detecting the conditions for which it was ordained—pre-eclampsia and intra-uterine-growth retardation—than a much more refined system that is being increasingly utilized.[7,23] By reducing the number of attendances, numbers at clinics are smaller and for those attending the atmosphere is much more leisurely and dignified. More time becomes available for those in greatest need, in particular the socially deprived, the grand multipara, the sick mothers, the teenage pregnancies, and the single-parent families. Reference to Tables 7.5, 7.6, 7.7, and 7.8 shows the great reductions in doctor and midwife

Table 7.5 *'New-style' obstetric programme for primigravida, 8–32 weeks*

Gestation in weeks	Done by	Major reasons
8	Midwife and doctor	Customary antenatal booking system
12	Midwife	Going along OK? Any questions . . .? Any more questions?
16		Scan at hospital.
22	Midwife	Baseline weight, blood-pressure, twins. Literature package (late pregnancy and labour) Arrangements for classes, films, NCT, etc.
26	Midwife	Weight, blood-pressure, reiterate literature, classes, etc.
30	Midwife and doctor	Assess foetal size, blood-pressure, weight, (predictive IUGR, pre-eclampsia). Customary blood-tests.

Table 7.6 *'New-style' obstetric programme for primigravida, 34–42 weeks*

Gestation in weeks	Done by	Major reasons
34	Midwife and doctor	Presentation. Pelvic assessment, blood-pressure, urine.
36	Midwife and doctor	Blood-pressure, urine, and presentation. Build up rapport, confidence. Discuss labour plan. Literature package (infant care).
	Family-planning nurse	Discuss contraception.
38	Midwife and doctor	As for 36 weeks (excluding literature and contraception). Engagement of presenting part.
40	Midwife and doctor	As for 38 weeks.
41	Midwife and doctor	As for 38 weeks. Confirm normality.
42	Midwife and doctor	As for 41 weeks. Double-check dates.

Table 7.7 *'New-style' obstetric programme for multipara, 8–32 weeks*

Gestation in weeks	Done by	Major reasons
8–12	Midwife and doctor	Customary antenatal booking system.
16		Scan at hospital.
22	Midwife	Baseline weight, blood-pressure, twins. Literature package (late pregnancy and labour). Arrangements for classes, films, National Childbirth Trust, etc.
30	Midwife and doctor	Assess foetal size. Blood-pressure, weight (predictive IUGR, pre-eclampsia). Customary blood-tests.

Table 7.8 *'New-style' obstetric programme for multipara, 34–42 weeks*

Gestation in weeks	Done by	Major reasons
36	Midwife and Doctor	BP, urine, and presentation. Build up rapport, confidence. Discuss labour plan. Literature package (infant care). Discuss contraception.
40	Midwife and doctor	As for 36 weeks (excluding literature and contraception). Engagement of presenting part.
41	Midwife and doctor	As for 40 weeks. Confirm normality.
42	Midwife and doctor	As for 41 weeks. Double-check dates.

care now appropriate for normal mothers in modern antenatal care. The 'major' reasons spelled out in the tables are discussed in greater detail elsewhere.[24] The point to be stressed here is the way that care is shared and reduced. By the same token, reference to Table 7.9 shows that the programme of postnatal care by the doctor is greatly curtailed. In the past, doctors made daily visits to their 'lying in' patients, whereas nowadays these mothers are busily up and about, and receiving continuing care from the midwife and, later, the health-visitor. Implicit in this 'new style'

Table 7.9   *'New-style' obstetric programme from labour to 6 weeks*

New style	Done by	Major reasons
1st stage	Midwife and doctor	Doctor provides continuity and confirms normality. Instills confidence into woman and companion. Supports midwife, deals with minor abnormalities. Decides on referral
2nd stage	Midwife and doctor	As above, doctor provides second pair of skilled hands
3rd stage	Midwife and doctor	As above. Scores bonding. Checks baby.
Day 1	Midwife and doctor	Checks baby.
Days 2–10 (at home)	Midwife	Daily care
Day 6	Midwife and doctor	Comprehensive baby check.
10 days to 6 weeks	Health-visitor	
6 weeks	Midwife and Doctor	Pelvic history and examination Cervical cytology
	Family-planning nurse	Preconception counselling. Contraception. Baby check, immunization programme

antenatal and postnatal care is that, if midwife or health-visitor detect problems, the doctor can be contacted.

Table 7.9 also describes the doctor's presence at every stage of labour and the reason for it. This involvement is much greater than in earlier years when mother and midwife were just 'left to get on with it'. Here is a good example of the expanded care of the doctor, at what is now seen as a very critical time in the mother's and baby's life; and this increased effort is possible because of other reductions in care that the doctor has made and that are being spelled out throughout this book.

Well-woman clinics

Well-woman clinics probably owe their growth in the last thirty years to the discovery of the cervical smear. Initially many of them were set up in the community under the auspices of the district health authority. Increasingly, general practices have a well-woman clinic, and their presence received further impetus from the orientation on prevention embodied in the 'new contract'.[8] All-important, however, is that the well-woman clinic is conducted by the practice nurse.

When the practice nurse sees the patient, she has her medical records available and can make some general enquiries about the patient's well-being and any current health problems. She orientates particularly on the menstrual history and then considers more general aspects of health, height/weight ratio, smoking, exercise, and so on. The protocol is described in Table 7.10. Attendance at such a clinic takes place every three years, coinciding with the recall date for routine cervical smear. A registered nurse is trained to use medical records, take relevant histories, and carry out breast and abdominal examinations. In my practice, our first nurse had not used the vaginal speculum for taking cervical smears. Accordingly, she was instructed on how to use it and she and the doctor who trained her took many cervical smears together and inspected many cervixes. She was provided with the relevant books and articles from the library of the local postgraduate centre.

Although initially the response from patients when sent for to attend well-women clinics was disappointing, in recent years it has become much more enthusiastic. The major findings are problems with weight, symptomless Trichomonas infection, detected coincidentally on a cervical smear, some minor abnormalities of the menstrual cycle, smokers, and hypertension. Only a small proportion of patients do require referral to the doctor for medical help. Although there is very little immediate return from such clinics apart from the occasional diagnostic discovery (maturity-onset diabetes, hypertension, and so on), it is the height/weight ratio and the counselling about exercise, hobbies, and the encouragement of more intellectual activities that probably in the long term benefit the women most and reduce their medical needs.

Well-man clinic

Table 7.11 shows the protocol which the nurse uses when running a well-man clinic. It is not dissimilar to the protocol for the well-woman clinic. Initially this clinic was badly attended, but as the British community as a whole is realizing the value of preventative care, men are beginning to come. They are advised to attend every five years after the age of 25. As with women, only very few men require doctor referral, and the major problems detected are obesity, smoking, lack of exercise, hypertension, and heavy drinking.[25]

New-patient clinic

All newly registering patients complete a proforma at the reception desk. Children under 16, adult females, and adult males have different forms

Table 7.10   *Well-woman clinic protocol*

Target Population: All women aged 16 to 74 inclusive

Protocol

Note: Age
Previous significant illnesses and operations
Occupation (and previous 'risk' occupations)
Smoking habits (now and previously)
Drinking habits (now and previously)
Family history of 'genetic' illnesses (e.g. diabetes, thyroid
disease, etc.)
Physical exercise
Mental exercise

Measure: Height
Weight
Sitting blood-pressure (diastolic at 5th Korotkov sound)—
compare with 'norm' for age
Peak-flow ratio for smokers—compare with norm for age

Test: Post-prandial urine for albumin and sugar
Haemoglobin if tired or pale
Triglycerides and cholesterol if significant family history
Other blood-tests   if specifically indicated
ECG
Chest X-ray

Discuss/advise on: Appropriate weight for height/nutrition (diet sheet)
Smoking and alcohol consumption (pamphlet)
Physical exercise
Mental exercise (courses, etc.)
Tetanus status (booster approximately 5-yearly or
commence a course)
Blood-pressure checks—if raised, check twice at different
times of day. If persistently raised and/or bad family
history, check triglycerides and cholesterol and then refer
to GP
Breast cancer and self examination
Cervical cancer and cytology—offer smear if necessary

Agree further management of any problems including referral to GP if necessary;
set review date as appropriate. If all well, routine repeat-attendance every three
years.

(Figures 7.2, 7.3, and 7.4). They are then advised to attend the practice
nurse's 'new-patient clinic'. If this can be preceded by a general 'wander'
around the practice premises accompanied by an informed receptionist, or
in some cases a 'front-office manager', so much the better. The nurse's

Table 7.11   *Well-man clinic protocol*

Target Population:	All men aged 16 to 74 inclusive
Protocol	
Note:	Age
	Previous significant illnesses and operations
	Occupation (and previous 'risk' occupations)
	Smoking habits (now and previously)
	Drinking habits (now and previously)
	Family history of 'genetic' illnesses (e.g. diabetes, thyroid disease, etc.)
	Physical exercise
	Mental exercise
Measure:	Height
	Weight
	Sitting blood-pressure (diastolic at 5th Korotkov sound)—compare with 'norm' for age
	Peak-flow ratio for smokers—compare with norm for age
Test:	Post-prandial urine for albumin and sugar
	Haemoglobin if tired or pale
	Triglycerides and cholesterol if significant family history
	Other blood-tests if specifically indicated
	ECG
	Chest X-ray
Discuss/advise on:	Appropriate weight for height/nutrition (diet sheet)
	Smoking and alcohol consumption (pamphlet)
	Physical exercise
	Mental exercise (courses, etc.)
	Tetanus status (booster approximately 5-yearly or commence a course)
	Blood-pressure checks—if raised, check twice at different times of day. If persistently raised and/or bad family history, check triglycerides and cholesterol and then refer to GP
	Testicular cancer and self examination

Agree further management of any problems including referral to GP if necessary; set review date as appropriate. If all well, routine repeat-attendance every five years.

main role is to ensure that children's immunizations have been completed and developmental paediatric checks are up to date. The 'new contract' has given added impetus to this. Shortcomings in immunization can be corrected, and developmental checks can be directed to the health visitor. As far as adults are concerned, the nurse can run through the protocol for

Norton Medical Centre
Harland House
Norton

Details of Children (under 16) living at your address and registering with our Practice

	Child 1	Child 2	Child 3
NAME	....	....	....
SEX	....	....	....
DATE OF BIRTH	....	....	....

**Please tick if your child has
had the following immunisations
and give dates if possible:**

	Child 1	Child 2	Child 3
1st Triple Diphtheria/Tetanus/Polio	....	....	....
1st Pertussis (Whooping Cough)	....	....	....
2nd Triple Diphtheria/Tetanus/Polio	....	....	....
2nd Pertussis (Whooping Cough)	....	....	....
3rd Triple Diphtheria/Tetanus/Polio	....	....	....
3rd Pertussis (Whooping Cough)	....	....	....
MMR or Measles	....	....	....
Pre-school Booster	....	....	....
Rubella (German Measles)	....	....	....

**Does your child suffer from any
medical problems such as diabetes,
asthma, etc?**

	Child 1	Child 2	Child 3
	yes/no details:	yes/no details:	yes/no details:
	....	....	....
	....	....	....

**If so, does he/she take any
prescribed medicine?**

	Child 1	Child 2	Child 3
	yes/no details:	yes/no details:	yes/no details:
	....	....	....
	....	....	....

Fig. 7.2.   New-patient form: child under 16

Norton Medical Centre
Harland House
Norton

NEW PATIENT-FEMALE over 16 years

Welcome to our Practice! We will request your medical records from your previous doctor, but there is often a delay before they arrive — sometimes up to three months. We need some information to be able to care for you in the meantime, so please take a few minutes to fill out this form.

Additionally, if you have not had a check-up in the last year — or would just like to know more about our facilities — please ask the Receptionist for a New Patient Appointment.

FULL NAME: ....

ADDRESS: ....

....

PHONE NO: ....

DATE OF BIRTH ....

Have you recently been attending your doctor's surgery for regular checks or a current problem?
Yes/No

If so, please give details: ....

....

Do you have any tablets, medicines or inhalers prescribed for you?   Yes/No

If so, please give details: ....

....

Please tick the appropriate box if you or your parents have suffered any of the following:

	Self	Father	Mother
Diabetes			
High Blood Pressure/Stroke			
Asthma			
Heart Problems			
Thyroid Problems			

Have you had a hysterectomy?   Yes/No

If not, a) do you currently take the Pill? If so, which one?   ....

b) do you have a coil fitted? If so, when was it fitted?   ....

c) If you are between 20 and 65 years old, when did you last have a cervical smear?   ....

Fig. 7.3. New patient form: female over 16

Norton Medical Centre
Harland House
Norton

NEW PATIENT-MALE over 16 years

Welcome to our Practice!   We will request your medical records from your previous doctor, but there is often a delay before they arrive — sometimes up to three months. We need some information to be able to care for you in the meantime, so please take a few minutes to fill out this form.

Additionally, if you have not had a check-up in the last year — or would just like to know more about our facilities — please ask the Receptionist for a **New Patient Appointment.**

FULL NAME: ....

ADDRESS: ....

....

PHONE NO: ....

DATE OF BIRTH   ....

Have you recently been attending your doctor's surgery for regular checks or a current problem?
Yes/No

If so, please give details: ....

....

Do you have any tablets, medicines or inhalers prescribed for you?   Yes/No

If so, please give details: ....

....

Please tick the appropriate box if you or your parents have suffered any of the following:

	Self	Father	Mother
Diabetes			
High Blood Pressure/Stroke			
Asthma			
Heart Problems			
Thyroid Problems			

Fig. 7.4. New-patient form: male over 16

her well-man or well-woman clinic (see above). Elderly patients will be similarly checked, and the elderly-care visitor can call at their homes if they wish (see next section).

Elderly preventative care

There are a large number of services available to the elderly in the community, but many are unknown to their doctors. Domiciliary hairdressing, chiropody, meals on wheels, and library services are four examples. Working from a check-list, an elderly-care visitor can discuss these with patients and make appropriate arrangements. Such a service was provided in my practice three or four years ago, and was funded by an employment training grant.[20] It generated enormous satisfaction amongst our elderly patients and resulted in a protocol and a computer 'screen' for our future elderly-care visitors to use. Figure 7.5 shows the screen. The headings down the side are self-explanatory and it merely remains for the elderly-care visitors to insert appropriate code-numbers for a picture of that elderly person in their home to emerge. By plugging gaps in their care, much benefit will accrue to elderly patients. Although many of these benefits are social, their provision can be termed preventative care, and there is virtually no doctor involvement.

Adult-vaccination clinic

World travel increases and patients require various vaccinations. The practice nurse has a detailed map, and charts showing which vaccinations are required when visiting particular parts of the world. Travellers are advised by receptionists, or other team members, that the practice nurse is the expert and will organize an appropriate programme of vaccinations according to the individual traveller's needs. The programme takes cognizance of interactions between vaccines, and aims to minimize the side-effects and maximize the length of immunity. The nurse is aware of the problems of storage, shelf-life, sterilization of equipment, and so on. The regulations and clinical data change for various vaccinations from time to time, and she keeps up to date. At the bottom of Table 7.2 is a list of the vaccines that adults should receive. Influenza usually proves to be most contentious *vis-à-vis* practice policy. In my practice influenza vaccination 'on demand' is discouraged, and it is saved for the elderly in closed communities (such as old-people's homes), the chronic sick (diabetic, heart-failure, bronchitis, and so on), and health-care workers. The practice nurse, community nurse, health-visitor, and other 'paramedics' in the team seem to get their 'flu vaccinations regularly; the doctors seem to opt out! Even at the level of recipient, GPs are not good at preventative care: QED!

EC]Elderly Care   Patient No.[   ]

Name/Address   . . . .   age . . . .

Date of Consultation   [   ]   Review Date [   ] PHB

Home Accommodation   [   ] :

Coping Summary Code [   ]   :

GENERAL HEALTH   90   89   88   87   ACTION
Mobility   [   ] [   ] [   ] [   ] [   ]

Social   [   ] [   ] [   ] [   ] [   ]

Mood   [   ] [   ] [   ] [   ] [   ]

Vision   [   ] [   ] [   ] [   ] [   ]

Hearing   [   ] [   ] [   ] [   ] [   ]

Housing   [   ] [   ] [   ] [   ] [   ]

Continence   [   ] [   ] [   ] [   ] [   ]

Feet   [   ] [   ] [   ] [   ] [   ]

TOTAL

O.T. [   ]   Meals on Wheels [   ]   Home Help [   ]   Allowances [   ]   Stairs [   ]

CONTACTS   NAME   RELATIONSHIP   TELEPHONE
            [   ] [   ] [   ]
            [   ] [   ] [   ]
DATE VISIT OFFERED   [   ]   REFUSED   [   ]

Fig. 7.5.   Elderly-care screen

ADVERTISING PREVENTATIVE CARE

British people are increasingly aware of the need for preventative care, and the fact that facilities are available in many general practices. Some now come to their doctors asking for 'check-ups', or with a list of items that concern them—'my cholesterol', a 'heart check', a 'blood-pressure check', and so on. The efficient practice will try to accommodate and hence pre-empt this in various ways:

1. Newly registering patients should be made aware that preventative care is very much the job of the practice and that there are various provisions for it. This can be checked by an informed receptionist or when they see the practice nurse for their 'new-patient protocol'.

2. The waiting-room should have notices about the various preventative-care clinics, the times that they are run, who runs them—nurses, health-visitors, and so on—and the fact that the receptionist is the signpost to them and can make appropriate appointments. The 'in-house' notice-board of the efficient primary health-care team is of increasing importance.

3. Many practices now produce a brochure (see Chapter 14).[26,27] A study in my own practice showed that patients given a practice brochure used the services of the practice in a more appropriate way than those who were not given one.[28] The brochure should contain page-by-page accounts of the various preventative-care clinics available, the reasons for them, what to expect on attendance, when they are held, and who carries them out. Brochures initially were given only to patients of the practice, but now that advertising restrictions have been reduced by the General Medical Council many practice brochures will be available from the Family Health Services Authority, libraries, and post offices so that people in the community can learn of the differing facilities in practices.

4. To supplement the practice brochure, which is normally produced and revised only every few years, practices can publish newsletters with more month-by-month information. Any new clinics that have been organized or changes in the present ones can be described.

5. Leaflets about various preventative-care procedures, for example a leaflet on 'looking after your heart', may have a note attached indicating that the well-man or well-woman clinic is concerned with this, and encouraging patients to make appointments.

6. The practice annual report will contain a summary of the clinics and the numbers attending.[29] Perhaps, as audit increases, the amount of pathology that has been detected at such clinics will be included.

RECORDS AND COMPUTERS

The White Paper and the 'new contract' threw general practice into turmoil. Out of it is emerging one certainty: general practitioners will have to be computerized within the next few years in order to cope with the increased services they must provide. The efficient practice will have all its preventative care on computers, which will be programmed so that recalls for patients requiring family-planning checks, five-yearly well-man checks, three-yearly well-woman checks (including the cervical smear), and even ten-year checks for vaccinations such as tetanus, to name only a few, will all become part and parcel of an efficient, organized, computerized practice. Currently, some practices are still using various forms of card-index, or hand sorting of records, which, although reasonably effective, will be too cumbersome and too labour-intensive in the future. Transfer to computer is becoming mandatory. Increasingly, the secretarial, reception, and filing-clerk staff of the practice will become computer-access personnel. Certainly, in the efficient practice, each doctor will have a terminal on his desk which will, at the tap of the appropriate key, illuminate the preventative-care programme of the patient sitting in his consulting-room and highlight any deficiencies in it. Thus will opportunistic screening be facilitated, and the results immediately recorded for instantaneous updating. This is not a fantasy: some practices are doing it already.

PROBLEM PATIENTS—THE AWKWARD SQUAD

The deprived

The Black Report highlighted the differences in health between the social classes in Great Britain.[30] These differences between rich and poor—to put it in simplistic terms—are well known to every general practitioner. In a study in our own practice, we substantiated the conclusions of the Black Report and nowhere more so than in the field of preventative health.[4] The immunization rate, cervical cytology, blood-pressure checks, and attendances at well-person clinics were all significantly lower for social classes 4 and 5, compared with social classes 1 and 2. And yet it was amongst social classes 4 and 5 that preventative care was most needed. As a result, a 'blitz' was carried out in the most deprived area in our practice using the following five methods:

1. marking every deprived patient's record with the membership of the whole household to which they belonged and alongside them the preventative care that had been completed. Hence there was opportunity to update, or at least advise about the updating, of every member of the household even though perhaps only one member consulted;

2. giving copies of these household cards to health-visitors so that they could advise about appropriate procedures whenever they visited them;

3. getting the practice nurse to fit these patients in, whenever they attended the surgery; the data showed that as a group they were not good at keeping appointments;

4. the entire team, and especially the reception staff, were aware of this 'blitz' and directed attending family members to the practice nurse whenever an opportunity arose;

5. each household was written to twice within a period of six months, indicating which members required which item of preventative care.

As a result of these measures, the preventative-health gap between the deprived community, and an age/sex-matched control group in a nearby area, disappeared.[31,32] There is no doubt that a great deal more effort is required to get full preventative care carried out in deprived communities, but much of this work can be done by reception and records staff linking with the nursing members of the team; doctor involvement can be minimal.

The handicapped

Another group who require extra effort and probably do involve the doctor are the handicapped at home, whose immunizations, cervical cytology, and other checks are frequently lacking. It seems surprising at first sight that a woman totally paralysed from muscular dystrophy, and totally dependent on her husband, is still anxious that her cervical smear should be carried out; yet that was true in my own practice. Accordingly, nurses occasionally have to visit in the community to carry out such procedures. In the efficient practice this work is shared amongst the team members so the doctor's part in the care can be minimal. Occasionally he has to do immunizations in the house, or at least be there, for medico-legal reasons, if the nurse gives them.

RUNNING AT A PROFIT

Many practices have found that when there was automatic 70 per cent reimbursement of nurse salaries, then the amount of money generated on fee-for-service payments more than paid for the 30 per cent that the doctor had to find.[25,33] Indeed, in our practice so great were the numbers of immunizations and cervical smears that the fees exceeded the nurse's entire salary. Accordingly, when the work-load of the nurse became too great, we were able to employ a second practice nurse without any financial anxieties. Bear in mind, though, that the most cost-effective way of doing much of this work is to persuade the district health authority attached staff, currently still provided free for the practice, to do as much of this preventative work as possible. With their future uncertain, they seem increasingly willing to undertake these tasks.

MEDICO-LEGAL CONSIDERATIONS

Health-visitors, midwives, and community-nursing sisters are well aware of the degree of legal cover that they have from their employing district health authority. For the most part they are not prepared to exceed this, and rightly so. Accordingly, doctors need have few worries about the medico-legal side of these people's work, although this does mean from time to time that they will not be prepared to undertake duties which patently are well within their competence but unfortunately carry medico-legal dangers. A simple example is a community-nursing sister not being prepared to give 'flu vaccine or other preventative care immunizations in the homes of patients without a doctor present.

Practice nurse

It is the practice nurses, employed by the doctor, whose medico-legal cover has to be safeguarded.[34–36] Most of them continue membership of, or rejoin, the Royal College of Nursing which automatically provides them with medico-legal cover. The document *The Duty and Position of the Nurse* contains a statement jointly agreed by the British Medical Association and the Royal College of Nursing, and there is nothing in that statement that precludes the type of consultations carried out in well-person clinics. In addition, the practice nurse can carry out all injections, in either therapeutic or preventative fields, so long as there is a doctor in the building. She has ready-set trays with adrenalin, airways, and other emergency-care necessities, so that if there is a 'collapse' she has instant access to everything necessary, as well as instant access to a doctor. There must be a 'hot-line' in every practice, by which the practice nurse can summon a doctor immediately to her patient. The last time I was 'summoned' I delivered a baby!

Practice family-planning nurse

To the best of my knowledge, the medico-legal defensibility of a practice nurse carrying out family-planning consultations has never been tested in court. However, the doctors in our practice do not feel particularly at risk of litigation, nor does the nurse, because of the medico-legal cover provided by her membership of the Royal College of Nursing.

There is no doubt that the main defence of nurses, should untoward events occur, would be that they have been adequately trained for the task they are doing, have taken all necessary precautions, and have medical cover available immediately.

PREVENTATIVE CARE FROM THE PATIENT'S POINT OF VIEW

The ground-swell of opinion currently in the British community is that preventative care should be undertaken more commonly, and this concept has been fostered by the government in the recent White Paper and the 'new contract' for general practitioners. Increasingly, patients are asking for it. They want their preventative care convenient to their own home (for example, in their nearby surgery or medical centre); they want it at times that suit themselves, including evenings and Saturday mornings for working people; the female population would prefer it to be done by a woman,[37] and both sexes wish to be able to decline preventative care if they feel like it. They also wish not to burden doctors with what they perceive as trivial questions about their health. Accordingly, the principle of having preventative care carried out by nurses appeals to people very much. Certainly, our experience in our own practice is that preventative care from nurses is extremely well received, and seems very appropriate to the opinion-forming middle-class patients of the practice who increasingly flow in to receive it.

REFERENCES

1. Hart, J. T. (1987) *Hypertension: community control of high blood pressure*, 2nd edn. Churchill Livingstone, Edinburgh and London.
2. Hart, J. T., Stilwell, B., and Muir Gray J. A. (1988). *Prevention of coronary heart disease and stroke*. Faber, London.
3. Allen, I. (1988). *Doctors and their careers*. Policy Studies Institute, London.
4. Marsh, G. N. and Channing, D. M. (1986). Deprivation and health in one general practice. *British Medical Journal*, **292**, 1173–6.
5. Tinson, S. (1985). Supervision of mother and baby from 2 to 6 weeks. In Marsh, G. N. (ed.) *Modern obstetrics in general practice*. Oxford University Press.
6. Royal College of Midwives (1987). *Report on the role and education of the future midwife in the United Kingdom*. RCM, London.
7. Marsh, G. N. (1985). New programme of antenatal care in general practice. *British Medical Journal*, **291**, 644–8.
8. Marsh, G. N. (1976). Further nursing care in general practice. *British Medical Journal*, **2**, 626–7.
9. Marsh, G. N. (1985). Pre-conception counselling. In Marsh, G. N. (ed.) *Modern obstetrics in general practice*, Oxford University Press.
10. Dunnell, K. and Dobbs, J. (1982). *Nurses working in the community*. HMSO, London.
11. Baker, G., Bevan, J. M., McDonnell, L., and Wall, B. (1987). *Community nursing. Research and development*. Croom Helm, London.

12. Fowler, G., Fullard, E., and Gray, J. A. M. (1988). The extended role of practice nurses in preventive health care. In Bowling A. and Stilwell, B. (eds.) *The nurse in family practice*. Scutari, London.
13. Cater, L. and Hawthorn, P. (1988). Survey of practice nurses in the UK— their extended roles. In Bowling, A. and Stilwell, B. (eds.) *The nurse in family practice*. Scutari, London.
14. Stilwell, B. and Drury, M. (1988). Description and evaluation of a course for practice nurses. *Journal of the Royal College of General Practitioners*, **38**, 203–6.
15. Bowling, A. (1988). The changing role of the practice nurse in the UK—from doctor's assistant to collaborative practitioner. In Bowling, A. and Stilwell, B. *The nurse in family practice*. Scutari, London.
16. English National Board (1990). *The Challenges of primary health care in the 1990s. A review of education and training for practice nursing*.
17. Royal College of General Practitioners (1968). *The practice nurse*. Reports from general practice No. 10. RCGP, London.
18. Stanley, I. (1989). The nurse partner. *Practice Nurse*, **1**, 432–3.
19. Lee, T. (1989). Project 2000: a nursing revolution. *Update*, **39**, 449–50.
20. Hall, R. G. P. (1991). The health of the elderly. Unpublished thesis. Birmingham University.
21. Hall, D. M. B. (ed.) (1989). *Health for all children*. Oxford University Press.
22. Morrell, D. C. (1985). The final postnatal examination. In Marsh, G. N. (ed.) *Modern obstetrics in general practice*. Oxford University Press.
23. Hall, M. H. (1985). The antenatal programme. In Marsh, G. N. (ed.) *Modern obstetrics in general practice*. Oxford University Press.
24. Marsh, G. N. (1985). 'New style' obstetric care. In Marsh, G. N. (ed.) *Modern obstetrics in general practice*. Oxford University Press.
25. Marsh, G. N. and Chew, C. (1984). Well-man clinic in general practice. *British Medical Journal*, **288**, 200–1.
26. Mead, M. (1990). How to produce a practice leaflet. *Update*, **40**, 137–40.
27. British Medical Association (1986). *General practitioner services: GMSC's guidelines on practice booklets*. BMA, London.
28. Marsh, G. N. (1984). *Norton Medical Centre. A practice brochure*. MSD, Norton.
29. Gray, D. J. P. (1985). Practice annual reports in *The medical annual* (ed. D. J. P. Gray). Wright, Bristol.
30. Black Report (1980). *Inequalities in health*. DHSS, London.
31. Marsh, G. N. and Channing, D. M. (1988). Narrowing the health gap between a deprived and an endowed community. *British Medical Journal*, **296**, 173–6.
32. Marsh, G. N. and Channing, D. M. (1987). Comparison in use of health services between a deprived and an endowed community. *Archives of Disease in Childhood*, **62**, 392–6.
33. Wilson, D. (1988). How much is your practice nurse worth? *Medical Monitor*, **1**, (33):6.
34. Royal College of Nursing (1990). *Practice nursing: your questions answered*. RCN, London.
35. Schutte, P. (Winter 1990). The practice nurse. *Journal of the Medical Defence Union*, London.

36. Nutley, P. (1990). Are you liable for your practice nurse? *Medical Monitor*, London.
37. Nichols, S. (1987). Women's preferences for sex of doctor: a postal survey. *Journal of Royal College of General Practitioners*, **37**, 540–3.

8. Personal lists

One of the major complaints by patients about the grouping of doctors together in large practices is the inability to see the same doctor each time they consult.[1] Care given by a different doctor for each episode of illness seems unpopular; continuing, comprehensive, one-patient/one-doctor care seems to be appreciated.[2,3,4] People like to feel that they have their own doctor who has their best interests at heart and looks after them in a continuous way. When they do have a personal doctor, trust builds up over the years between doctor, patient, and also with the patient's family. There is no doubt that treating one member of a family well benefits the entire family. Perhaps one of the most 'bonding' things that a doctor can do is to attend a birth in the family, especially where the father is present too.[5] As years pass by the baby of that family is cared for by the doctor until she becomes a mature woman, and in turn the same doctor can be present when she delivers.[6]

This sort of relationship, a feature of long-established older doctors in the practice, facilitates efficient care. Where patient and doctor know each other in such a continuous way, care, whether it be psychological, emotional, or clinical, can be highly organized and cost-effective in time. It is obviously impossible for one doctor in a large group practice of, say, 10 000 or 20 000 patients—and such practices are becoming increasingly common—to know all the patients well. However, he can certainly know his own personal list of around 3000. By being on a personal list, and seeing the same doctor, the patients know his system, the way he works, and can use his skills appropriately. As an example, if a doctor in a practice does not like to make home visits to patients with 'flu and upper-respiratory-tract infection, then the patients of that doctor increasingly accept that they must attend the surgery for such illnesses. Similarly, when a doctor does not prescribe antibiotics for upper-respiratory-tract infections, he can teach his patients why and they can understand and accept this. The personal list is a means of avoiding the confusion arising from different styles of care for the same sort of illness. A doctor with a personal list can record in the way he wants. He can also read his own notes even if he cannot read anyone else's! Diagnostic parameters are his and are understood by him. He can use his own nomenclature and utilize his own 'favourite' prescriptions. Above all, with personal lists the doctor can use the team in his own particular way, and patients can get to know and understand this. Personal lists facilitate repeat prescriptions and, increasingly importantly, telephone consultations. Duplication of care is avoided: one doctor takes one history, makes one examination, and orders one set of investigations. The system of multiple doctors duplicates and replicates all these components of clinical care.

Many illnesses repeat themselves in many episodes: depression, dyspepsia, irritable bowel, ingrown toe-nails, phobias, eczema, asthma, and backache, to name but a few. The continuing recurring care by the same doctor means a quicker assessment and management, largely based on earlier knowledge of previous episodes.

With a personal list there is need to provide adequate access. No point in proclaiming the virtues of patients having their own doctor if he is not available virtually every day. This concept was embraced in the 'new contract' for general practice; daily availability of each doctor is now almost mandatory and facilitates personal care.[7] In my own practice, consultation analysis showed that, despite six weeks holiday per year, two weeks study leave, and a one-in-five rota for evenings and weekends, 85 per cent of surgery attendances and 80 per cent of home visits were undertaken by the patient's own doctor.[8] More importantly, all the major illnesses of patients were seen by their own doctor, perhaps not always at the 'emergency' onset but certainly for early follow-up and continuing care thereafter.

Establishing a personal-list system is not inordinately difficult. It involves spending two or three days—in my own practice the best part of a long weekend—breaking down the record system according to various parameters. First, according to the handwriting of the doctor that appeared most frequently in the record. Secondly, by the name of the doctor to whom most of the hospital letters were addressed. Thirdly, and perhaps most importantly, from the receptionists' knowledge of which doctor looked after which patients. Most group practices do subscribe to the view that they do run personal lists, at least informally, so breaking the records down into the individual lists is not as difficult as it might appear at first sight. Once done, patients wishing to see their own doctor needed to say which particular doctor they looked upon as their own. If the record had been mis-filed—and about 5 per cent had—they were transferred to the appropriate doctor. The interesting exercise of counting up which doctor had how many patients took place a few weeks later. From then on it was possible to equalize lists by directing new patients who did not request a particular doctor (about 70 per cent of them) to the doctors with the smallest lists. The doctor with the largest list ceased taking such patients for about a year until numbers on the other lists had caught up.

The major problem of individual lists is the isolation of each doctor within his own practice. As a result, practice rota arrangements for evening, nights, weekends, and holidays become the customary way of partners being aware of each-other's performance. In addition, the meetings where patients' care is shared with other members of the team also give some insight. Latterly, the establishment of protocols for preventative clinics and certain types of illness are helping to standardize care. Increasing use of computers, including the design of standardized software, has also brought individual list-holders together and opened up their care to peer scrutiny. Latterly, practice educational programmes, especially ones recognized for the postgraduate educational allowance, can serve as an opportunity for cross-fertilization of ideas. Personal-list doctors with a trainee working alongside may need to create a certain amount of appointment 'hunger' to help receptionists persuade patients to consult the trainee. On the other hand, a personal list facilitates the trainer's teaching since he knows his patients well, and continuously, and hopefully understands their problems well. Trainers teach better on known patients. Personal lists facilitate audit and research, particularly since the 'denominator'—the number of patients—is known, and this is frequently needed for research projects. Audit of each doctor's work can generate interesting comparisons, one doctor to another, and league tables—often the subject of ribald comment—can emerge. Where there are other commitments outside the practice (such as paid clinical or administrative posts), reduction in individual lists can be organized so that work-loads can continue to be equalized. There is no doubt that organizing a personal list under the umbrella of the group produces one of the most economic systems of care, and the implementation and full fruition of many of the ideas in this book depend upon it.

PERSONAL LISTS FROM THE PATIENT'S POINT OF VIEW

Personal, continuing, one-doctor care is highly valued by patients. They do not like the contradictions that result from several general practitioners' opinions, nor do they accept confusion in the method of care or the therapy. Patients are prepared to make allowances for the inexactitude of general practice medicine especially when it is prescribed by someone they know and trust. As a safeguard against the 'not good' or 'not caring' doctor, or against the inevitable personality conflicts between patient and doctor, patients needs to be able to change their doctor freely, either within a practice or from one practice to another; this has been facilitated by the 'new contract'. Nevertheless, patients rarely seem to change their doctors, and it seems that the great majority of them settle into a relationship with one doctor and like to see it continuing.

REFERENCES

1. Tant, D. (1985). Personal lists. *Journal of the Royal College of General Practitioners*, **35**, 507–9.

2. Marsh, G. N. (1972). Controversial view: 'back to single-handed'. *RCGP North-east Faculty Newsletter*.
3. Gray, D. J. Pereira (1979). The key to personal care. *Journal of the Royal College of General Practitioners*, **29**, 666–78.
4. Freeman, G. (1985). Priority given by doctors to continuity of care. *Journal of the Royal College of General Practitioners*, **35**, 423–6.
5. Marsh, G. N. (1982). The 'specialty' of general practitioner obstetrics. *Lancet*, **1**, 669–72.
6. Marsh, G. N. and Channing, D. M. (1989). Audit of 26 years of obstetrics in general practice. *British Medical Journal*, **298**, 1077–80.
7. Department of Health (1989). Terms of service for doctors in general practice. London: DOH.
8. Marsh, G. N. (1974). Team workload in general practice. Unpublished MD thesis. University of Newcastle upon Tyne.

9. Practice boundaries and branch surgeries

PRACTICE BOUNDARIES

Under the terms of the 'new contract', each practice is expected to have a definite boundary which is known to patients, all members of the primary health-care team, and the Family Health Services Authority.[1] It is another way of facilitating efficient care, and many organized practices have had one for years. Despite earlier references to this topic when discussing home visiting (see Chapter 3), and at the risk of some repetition, I will now discuss it in some detail.

Despite the fact that home visits are dwindling, they still continue to be a fairly time-consuming feature of most practices in Great Britain—and rightly so (Chapter 3).[2,3] In bad weather and during 'flu epidemics the numbers of home visits grow. At such times, practices without practice boundaries and with distant patients experience great problems. On the whole, sicker patients tend not to change their doctor, and it is possible to have an increasingly sick population the further away it is from the practice premises. A home visit takes approximately four times as long as seeing a patient at the surgery; this factor increases the more distant the patient is. This is a problem, not only for the doctors but for any members of the team who carry out home visits—midwives, community nurses, health-visitors, elderly-care visitors, and the rest. In some areas patients live across FHSA boundaries, which introduces complication of registration, payment, and so on. District health authorities also have boundaries, and attached members of their staff may not be allowed to cross them. The ideal situation is where a practice has a tight geographical boundary within both FHSA and district-health-authority boundaries.

For the distant patient, getting to the surgery can be difficult. Long walks, changing buses, expensive fares, several busy roads to cross are all familiar problems. By the same token, team members have greater difficulty reaching distant patients, and this can be particularly problematic in an emergency. Where patients live a long way from the surgery, there is a natural reluctance for all team members to carry out follow-up home visits. Patients with angina, previous myocardial infarctions, severe asthma, or poorly controlled epilepsy need to be close to good medical centres. The socially deprived, and in particular those with large numbers of small children, also need a surgery nearby.

How to rationalise the practice geography and create a boundary is fairly straightforward. By sampling, say, one in ten of the patients' records it is possible to build up a picture, using flags or other markers, on a detailed street-map, of where the patients live. Usually they are found in clusters, and knowledge of the size of the clusters and their frequency in certain areas helps to determine where the practice boundary should be.[4] Cognizance can be taken of fast access roads, as well as barriers such as level crossings, bottle-necks, and so on. Once the practice boundary is agreed, it can be implemented by removing groups of patients 'little by little'. Letters can be written to, say, thirty or forty patients per week indicating that the practice can no longer visit the area in which they are living, and suggesting that they change their doctor to someone nearer their own home. This letter must contain an explanation as to why this is being done, coupled with an expression of regret. Doctors can add personal notes to particular patients on the bottom of the standard letter. In our own practice, we removed 800 patients from the list in groups of 200. The response was very good and the reasons well understood. Occasionally, however, doctors will be involved in consultations with patients seeking to remain on the list for many and varied reasons; one of the main ones is the fact that they have 'always come to this practice'. To uphold the democratic decision that has been made, and in the interests of the whole team's care, doctors have to insist that these patients do leave. Exceptions will, of course, be made for the dying, the very ancient, clinical colleagues—nurses, doctors, and so on—and occasionally for other social reasons. In such instances these patients should be brought to the notice of the whole team so that they know they exist and have been made exceptions. Their records can be appropriately marked.

In our own practice we decided on a definitive boundary, but also allowed some 'grey areas'. In these we did not remove the patients already on our lists but decided not to accept any new patients in such areas nor continue to care for any of our patients who moved to live in them. Little by little the practice population in the 'grey areas' has dwindled.

An interesting sequel to our geographical rationalization was its effect on neighbouring practices. They too began to rationalize their geography, and one or two of them decided not to look after patients near our own premises; hence, some of these patients registered with us. Although initially our list fell by about 800, it began to grow again fairly rapidly, but with patients who lived nearer.

It is now mandatory for the Family Health Services Authority to know practice boundaries and if these are to be altered they must be informed.

It is essential, if the practice boundary is to succeed, that all doctors comply. The team members too must all be aware of the practice boundary so that all say the same thing to patients. The receptionists, faced with anxious and sometimes irritated patients, need to know how they should go about finding another doctor. From time to time, at practice meetings, the boundary can be discussed. In addition, doctors can discuss occasional patients that they wish to continue to care for, even though they have moved outside the boundary. The necessity for such special pleading certainly limits the numbers!

As a result of tight practice boundaries, branch surgeries have decreased in value, a laudable side-effect of a geographically cost-effective practice.

BRANCH SURGERIES

The branch surgery is to some extent a relic from earlier, less organized times. Their provision can prove extremely uneconomical. Doctors, nurses, receptionists, and other staff are all required to run them as well as their main surgery, so duplication necessarily results. They are expensive with regard to capital costs and equipment, and telephone access can be a problem. Duplication of provision in this way drains the resources of the whole practice, and what frequently results are better facilities in the main surgery than are provided at the branch. Branch surgeries may well not contain items of more expensive equipment, such as ECG machines, and not have available resuscitation equipment. Nor will they necessarily provide the various clinics—well-person, paediatric surveillance, minor ops, diabetic, and so on—which are being encouraged under the terms of the 'new contract'.

They can also present problems with regard to patients' records, since the comprehensive 'folder', of whatever type, cannot simultaneously be present at the main centre and the branch surgery; yet from time to time patients will go to both places. To overcome this, some branch surgeries have a direct computer link with the main centre, but this is rare, and it is likely, in my view, that branch surgeries will close as efficiency increases rather than being 'updated' in such a way. Branch surgeries reflect the days when patients were far less mobile, but about 90 per cent of the community now have either their own transport or someone else's available to them, so the need for the branch surgery has accordingly diminished. In my own practice, the branch surgery was situated only three or four bus-stops on a main bus-route from the main medical centre. It had been put there in an attempt to recruit patients from a developing 'new town'. Having served this purpose, it closed in 1964. In spite of there being other main surgeries close to our branch, patients did not leave the practice but merely stayed on the bus, or drove, a little longer.

The importance of branch surgeries will vary from one practice to another, but in my visits around the country it has been apparent to me that many of them are perpetuating habits and provisions that are no longer cogent. Perhaps a case can still be made for branch surgeries in remote rural areas, but in urban areas their existence seems very questionable.

Where branch surgeries are of considerable significance and size, and yet far away from the main centre, it could be geographically logical to consider splitting into two major practices, with simultaneous attention to practice boundaries, and so on. The details of such practice cataclysms are beyond the scope of this book.

PRACTICE BOUNDARIES AND BRANCH SURGERIES FROM THE PATIENT'S POINT OF VIEW

On the whole, patients would prefer to live close to their doctor's surgery. Certainly, the pram-pushing parents of young children, and the elderly, look upon this as a definite bonus. If the practice boundary is reasonably tightly drawn, particularly in urban and suburban areas, then obviously such patients will live within easy access. In addition, it is helpful for patients to know what the practice boundary is, so that those who are particularly happy with their doctor and team can bear this in mind when moving house, and similarly, those who feel shortcomings in the system can take good care to move well outside!

As far as branch surgeries are concerned, patients increasingly expect the whole gamut of facilities when they attend a practice, and prefer them all to be under one roof. They are well aware when facilities in branch surgeries are minimal and are prepared to make a slightly greater effort to attend the better-equipped main ones. Just as people are aware of the updating and improvement of facilities in banks, building societies, solicitor's offices, and architects' rooms, so they expect better, brighter, and more comprehensive services when they attend their doctor. It is unlikely that branch surgeries can compete with this, and many of them could and should be closed. On balance, patients would lose very little.

REFERENCES

1. Department of Health (1989). *Terms of service for doctors in general practice.* DOH, London.
2. Marsh, G. N., McNay, R. A., and Whewell, J. (1972). Survey of home visiting by general practitioners in north-east England. *British Medical Journal*, **1**, 487–92.
3. Whewell, J., Marsh, G. N., and McNay, R. A. (1983). Changing patterns of home visiting in the north of England. *British Medical Journal*, **286**, 1259–61.
4. Baker, R. H. (1984). The patient map as an aid to surgery planning. *Practitioner*, **228**, 1085–7.

10. Efficient records and the switch to computers

There is no doubt that if at each patient–doctor contact a concise yet comprehensive record was immediately available then the flow and speed of the consultation would be facilitated. The first part of this chapter describes such a record system in a manual form. However, manual records are increasingly being transferred to computer, so later in this chapter a computerized system is outlined and its contribution to ever-greater efficiency emphasized. Since one of the main tasks of computerized systems is to embody all the best aspects of the manual record, a few paragraphs, which at first sight may appear a little dated, on the A4 folder versus FP5/6 record-envelope debate are included. They will also be useful for the few brave souls struggling against the tidal wave of modern technology who have decided not to computerize.

General practitioners who have practised for a considerable time and have kept comprehensive records, do find that many many patients have the same illness repeatedly across the years. They frequently experience the same complex of symptoms associated with their depression, or their urinary-tract infection, or their musculo-skeletal pains. Scanning back over easily read, well-ordered records frequently reveals to both doctor and patient exactly what the current illness is by virtue of the fact that the patient has had it before. Even more importantly the therapy used previously is spelled out, as well as the results it achieved. If it was successful then, it can be used again this time. An easy method of care—one I commend to my trainees when I emphasize the importance of the previous history—and extremely efficient.

A4 OR FP5/6 RECORDS

Over many years there has been continuing debate about the need for general practitioners to convert the standard DOH issue FP5/6 record envelopes to A4 folders. Despite many attempts to improve the FP5/6 envelope, including the use of various insert cards (database, family planning, obstetric, and so on) the envelopes have proved increasingly inadequate.[1,2] A4 folders offer more space for recording in general, the systematic placing of basic data, a summary of the patient's significant illnesses, usually on view opposite the day-to-day record, and most importantly space for other team members to record. These advantages have all been well documented.[3] Indeed, it was following much work at the then DHSS that the A4 folder and its inserts were designed, and these are the basis of many standard A4 folder systems in general practice.[4] Sadly the enthusiasm for them at the DHSS waned, the money ran out, and only a small proportion of general practitioners received them free of charge. Some bought A4 folders of their own, but this proved expensive and was unusual.[5,6]

How to convert the FP5/6 envelope to the A4 folder has been recorded in one seminal monograph.[7] This was used as the basis for the conversion in our own practice, and the results were described.[8] The existence of these and other papers precludes the need to describe the detail of the conversion.[6,9] Suffice to say, that one of the most important principles, and one particularly embodied in our own practice, was that virtually all the work was done by lay-people. Only initial surveys of other practices further ahead with A4 folders, and the general organization of how the work was to be carried out, was done by doctors. The actual change-over was done by a Fine Arts graduate supported by clerical staff. Indeed, attempts by doctors to do the conversion were always inferior to those by lay-people, whose interest, enthusiasm, and accuracy were greater.

The ideal manual record

On opening a patient's record at the beginning of the consultation, the day-to-day notes should be instantly available to the doctor. These notes should be concise—this is the record of a lifetime, so there is no room for more than a line or two for the great majority of minor episodes of illness, such as respiratory infection, diarrhoea, aches and pains, and the like. The writing should be readable. If the doctor's handwriting is not legible except to himself, at least at the end of each dated consultation should be a 'box' in which the diagnosis is printed. Hence on scanning the right-hand edge of the record there should be a list of legible diagnoses. Behind the clinical notes should be the date-ordered investigations—haematology, biochemistry, X-rays, and so on. Exactly opposite them, and again immediately visible, should be a summary of the important illnesses from which this patient has suffered (Fig. 10.1). Each practice can decide which illnesses are significant enough to be included in a summary, but obviously all serious conditions such as congestive heart failure, endogenous depression, and major operations would be included. Many of the illnesses on the summary sheet will be those for which patients will have been to hospital. The hospital letters must be date-ordered and can be behind the summary sheet. Drug allergies, sensitivities, and side-effects should be prominently featured. In the DHSS A4 issue there is a special sheet for these pasted immediately inside the folder. Below this are listed serially the patient's occupations across the years.

National Health Service Number		

SUMMARY OF IMPORTANT ILLNESSES AND INVESTIGATIONS

Surname (Block Letters)	Forenames (Block Letters)

Address	Date of Birth

Date	

FAMILY HISTORY	NIL	FATHER	MOTHER	SIBLING
DIABETES	✓			
THYROID DISEASE ...	✓			
GOUT	✓			
PERNIC. ANAEMIA ...	✓			
ISCHAEMIC HEART D. ...	✓			
STROKE OR HYPERT'N ...			✓	
BLINDNESS Glaucoma ...	✓			

Date	
1956	Hepatitis
1973	Anaemia
1977	Incisional hernia
1981	Sigmoidoscopy - diverticulae - rectal polyp
1984	Sterilisation
1985	Hypertension

Form FP111G

Fig. 10.1. Example of summary of patient's previous important illnesses.

With the increasing emphasis on prevention, records must contain detail of preventative care. In the DHSS A4 folder this is a buff-coloured sheet on which immunizations, cervical smears, and blood-pressure, urine, and weight checks are all itemized (Fig. 10.2). Hence there is a running account of changes in these measurements across the years. By adding 'rubber-stamped' headings to this sheet, running accounts of smoking habits, alcohol intake, hobbies, exercise, and the like can be collated, the data largely emanating from attendances at well-person clinics (Fig. 10.3).

Also included somewhere near the summary of important illnesses should be a concise family history (Fig. 10.1). In our own practice we include diabetes, thyroid disease, gout, pernicious anaemia, ischaemic heart disease, stroke and/or hypertension, and blindness (glaucoma). Alongside the family-history 'box' there is room left for family anecdotes that can be important: 'only son died on Everest expedition' or 'husband of the practice tea lady' are two important, yet wildly different, examples. More complicated family-history sheets are available, but the important underlying principle is that there should be at least something about the patient's family in every well-ordered record. In some practices, lay staff write on the front of the folder or envelope any information (particularly preventative care) which they see to be missing from the record, to highlight to the doctor, when a consultation takes place, that this needs updating.

Not only doctors write in records. There can be, and are in many systems, separate records for obstetrics, family-planning, and other special clinics such as vascular, diabetic, and menopause clinics. These records follow the lines of the protocols established for these conditions (see Chapter 7). Their place in the record must be agreed by all those who use it. It is often helpful if these records are in different colours; hence a vascular-clinic sheet can be on red paper, a diabetic sheet on green, and so on. Such simple measures all lead to rapidity of access, more comprehensive information and care, and greater efficiency.

Health-visitors keep their own records for the children in their care, but in some practices they are included within the full folder. They are available not only to the health-visitors when they consult, but also to the doctors or nurses who can see what the health-visitor has been dealing with when patients in turn consult them. Similarly, health-visitors can read what doctors, nurses, and others have been dealing with.

Uniformity

All doctors must try to record in a standard fashion. It is well worth holding several team meetings to discuss how this difficult step can be taken. Compromise has to be the order of the day. In my own practice, there is now a clause in the practice agreement which states: 'The partners shall at all times . . . keep a proper record of every examination of every

	National Health Service Number	

	Surname (Block Letters)	Forenames (Block Letters)
IMMUNISATIONS AND SCREENING INVESTIGATIONS		
	Address	Date of Birth

IMMUNISATIONS (Insert date where appropriate)

	Diphtheria	Pertussis	Tetanus	Polio	Measles	Rubella	TAB	Smallpox
1			Refused					
2								
3								
Boost								
Boost								
Boost								

	Tuberculin Test				BCG.			
Result				Date				
Date								

Other Inoculations

Type								
Date								
Type								
Date								
Type								
Date								

SCREENING INVESTIGATIONS

Chest X-Ray (Date)	Cervical Smear (Date)	Blood Pressure			Urine			Miscellaneous		
		Date			Date	Albumen	Sugar	Date	Weight	Other (Specify)
1984 NAD	1977	1984	110/60		4.7.84	O	O	11.11.87	11 st	
	26.5.77	11.11.87	110/80							
	17.1.80									
	5.3.81									
	29.9.83									
	12.9.84									
	4.12.85									
	11.11.57									

SCREENING INVESTIGATIONS CONTINUED OVERLEAF

FORM FP 111 H

4509 Dd 8810849 366M 3/84 A G Ltd 52-0-0

Fig. 10.2.   DHSS A4 summary sheet: results and measurements

SCREENING INVESTIGATIONS Continued from overleaf

Chest X-Ray (Date)	Cervical Smear (Date)	Blood Pressure		Urine			Miscellaneous		
		Date		Date	Albumen	Sugar	Date	Weight	Other (Specify)

Other Procedures

Date		Date	CONTRACEPTIVE PRACTICE	Date	
					SMOKING
		1987	Sterilised	1987	10/day
		EXER			**RUBELLA STATUS**
		1987	Walking		HAD INFECTION ....
					HAS ANTIBODIES ....
					HAD INJECTION ....
					ALCOHOL
					1987 v. little
		HOBBIES			

Fig. 10.3 DHSS A4 summary sheet: summary of general information regarding patient

patient made by them and a sufficient note of the treatment or other remedy prescribed or advised and in such a way that any partner subsequently can continue care appropriately.'

This is the only clause in the whole agreement that mentions clinical standards. It emphasizes good record-keeping, and it is particular importance when various doctors may well be continuing care from one to the other. There should also be an in-house 'shorthand', and in my own such abbreviations as 'A' = attendance, 'V' = visit, 'T' = telephone consultation, 'D' = discussion without seeing the patient, are simple examples. Unnecessary words such as 'BP' or 'Temp' need not be included, since the figures that follow are self-evident.

Let me emphasize at the end of this section that all the date-ordering and organization of the record, once it is designed by the doctors, can be implemented by lay staff, and the clinical summaries similarly are done by them according to set protocols. The all-important principle is that all information is in the same place in every folder or card.

If lay-people really are involved in the records to the degree I have suggested, it should be eminently possible for them to complete the majority of the insurance medical forms, where the patient does not require to be seen by the doctor. All the doctor needs to do is to check over what has been written, and fill in certain 'starred' areas himself which may be problematic; the time saved can be considerable.

THE SWITCH TO COMPUTERS

Already some practices have put on to computer a large amount of the material currently in their manual records; indeed, much that I have described in the preceding paragraphs.[10–12] Many more are grinding through the long process of doing so. Most practices now have all their patients registered on a computer with their basic name, address, date of birth, telephone number, and other details. This at least provides them with an age/sex register. After the basic data, the most prevalent computer system is one that provides repeat prescribing.[13,14] Thus, many practices, even if they have no other form of computerization, are saving a large amount of receptionist and clerical time (see Chapter 6).

When doctors and members of the team have terminals on their desks, acute prescribing for the patient actually consulting them can be undertaken. It does necessitate room for a 'printer', but this can usually be accommodated close to the patient's hand, and its activation will serve as one indicator that the consultation is at an end! By using pre-programmed options for acute prescribing, the latter can become standardized, efficient, quick (quicker than handwriting, even with a pre-headed prescription), and most importantly, can incorporate the schedule of prescriptions ordained by the practice formulary or 'minicopoeia'.[15,16] Doctors will no longer be victims of the vagaries of their own memories and idiosyncracies, but will be presented with lists of options—for example, specific antibiotics and non-steroidal anti-inflammatory drugs—with the amounts and the dosage-schedule pre-ordained for the particular condition they have diagnosed. Further technological sophistication now allows the computer to prevent the prescription of drugs which interact, either those acute ones on the prescription currently being given, or the acute drug's interactions with 'repeat' medications that the computer already knows that the patient is taking. It should soon be possible for the computer to query the medication being prescribed if it seems inappropriate for the diagnosis that the doctor may have typed. For example, if a diagnosis of upper-respiratory tract infection has been made, it can query whether the antibiotics prescribed are appropriate and possibly request the 'complication' of the upper-respiratory-tract infection for which the antibiotics are indicated. Thus will 'big brother' begin to check up on a doctor's therapeutic work—many would say, all to the good. But an early major benefit of having all prescribing on the computer is the ability to audit what has been given and question its therapeutic efficiency.[16]

In the computerized consulting-room of the future, when the patient enters, the 'identification screen' will be illuminated. Let me presume it is the doctor who is consulting. If the patient is well known, the doctor will probably switch to his day-to-day clinical notes on the screen; he will add the recent history and findings, and sometimes make a diagnosis. This degree of keyboard-use may well mean that he will have to learn to type with more than two or three fingers—and certainly new entrants to general practice will find it worthwhile. Because in the great majority of practices the build-up of years' worth of clinical written notes and letters will be too large to be put into the computer, these will have to be available for a long time. This availability is particularly important if the principle I have enunciated earlier in this book is valid: that since everybody has had everything before, referral to previous episodes is extremely efficient in time and effort (see Chapter 4).

If the doctor does some preventative work—asks about smoking habits, checks blood-pressure and/or urine, for instance—then by pressing an appropriate key the preventative-care screen can be called up and the data entered, probably as quickly as writing it on preventative-care sheets.

Increasingly there will be various 'special screens' which can be called up by the doctor as appropriate. A family-history screen will be in every patient's notes and will occasionally have additions made to it. If the doctor wishes to review the diabetic care of a patient in front of him who is suffering from an inter-current illness, he can call up the diabetic screen. The screen for vascular disease will include histograms of changes of hypertension across the years. The physiotherapist's or dietitian's care can be provided on a screen. Every illness or preventative routine can lend itself to a protocol of care in the practice; these protocols can become screens on the VDU. Allergies, sensitivities, and side-effects will be on another screen, as will the details of preventative care in the other members of the household to which the patient belongs; hence an opportunity for promulgating household preventative care. Instead of the doctor flicking across record sheets, he will be flicking across computer screens. And as the patient leaves, it could well be that repeat appointments will be organized by computer at the reception desk.

Patchily, here and there across the surgeries of the country, computer facilities and efficiencies are proceeding, and this should lead to more efficient care. In the interim there may well be semi-'organized' chaos, but gradually the shift to computers should prove its worth, resulting in a better, quicker, more organized, and more retrievable system than the manual record could ever achieve. There will be no end to the opportunities for audit and even research; selection of *what* to do will increasingly be the problem.

THE 'COMPUTER ILLITERATES'—PEOPLE LIKE ME

Many doctors—and I have great sympathy with them—will not be able, or even will not wish, to share most of their consulting-time with their patient 'calling up' screens, reading illuminated text, and tapping computer keys. For them it should be possible for a trained clerk to be so familiar with the doctor's manual records that they can be retrieved after the consultation session and the appropriate pieces of information put into the computer. The screens on such doctors' desks would then serve as an up-to-date information system for them, without the doctors themselves being involved in the work. Such a system would also be invaluable for new entrants to the practice, or temporary people—locums, and so on—who would not be expected to be immediately computer-literate.

For those like me who believe the computer should be servant rather than taskmaster, I commend the above paragraph. And I can see greater overall accuracy of data from using trained records/computer clerks than from a plethora of clinicians with varying degrees of computer literacy and enthusiasm.

EFFICIENT RECORDS AND THE SWITCH TO COMPUTERS FROM THE PATIENT'S POINT OF VIEW

There is no doubt that, in my own practice, patients have shown great interest at each step of the records-improvement, from the old Lloyd

George envelope to the A4 folder, then to the computer database, and finally to computerized clinical notes. By showing them the various sheets inside the record, they have become aware that their care has become more comprehensive and more detailed and itemized. More recently they have become interested in looking at computer screens to see what is recorded; this can be encouraged; full access to records by patients is not far off; access to computer data is now mandatory by law.[17] However, patients need to be reassured of the security of the data just as they have been reassured in the past of the security of the record folders (more honoured in the intent than in the reality!).

Patients can have confidence that updating is taking place and that they will be recalled regularly for preventative measures. And by having a household screen, they can see that the doctor takes an interest in their entire family; they will be able to provide information about non-attending members. Having said all that, there is some anecdotal evidence that patients do not like their doctor puzzling over a VDU during their consultation with him. There has always been much complaint from patients about doctors, and particularly hospital doctors, consulting the records rather than consulting the patient. Will doctors of the future be accused of consulting the computer? Plainly there is much work and analysis to be done on the acceptability or otherwise of computer technology.

REFERENCES

1. Cormack, J. J. C. (1971). *The general practitioner's use of medical records.* Edinburgh Scottish Home and Health Department.
2. Cormack, J. J. C. (1970). The medical record envelope—a case for reform. *Journal of the Royal College of General Practitioners*, **20**, 333–53.
3. Department of Health and Social Security (1974). *Joint working party on re-design of medical records in general practice.* Interim report. HMSO, London.
4. Department of Health and Social Security (1978). *Second report of the joint working party on re-design of medical records in general practice.* HMSO, London.
5. Hawkey, J. K., London, I. S. L., Greenhalgh, G. P., and Bungay, G. T. (1971). New record folder for use in general practice. *British Medical Journal*, **4**, 667–70.
6. Elliott, A., Walker, G. H. D., and Brockis, R. J. (1975). Complete conversion of health centre medical records to A4 size. *British Medical Journal*, **4**, 773–4.
7. Zander, L. I., Beresford, S. A. A., and Thomas, P. (1978). *Medical records in general practice.* Occasional Paper No. 5. RCGP, London.
8. Marsh, G. N. and Thornham, J. R. (1980). Changing to A4 folders and updating records in a 'busy' general practice. *British Medical Journal*, **281**, 215–17.

9. Acheson, H. W. K. (1976). Converting medical records to A4 size in general practice. *Journal of the Royal College of General Practitioners*, **26**, 277–81.
10. Bradshaw-Smith, J. H. (1976). A computer record-keeping system for general practice. *British Medical Journal*, **1**, 1395–7.
11. Preece, J. F. and Hearson, J. R. (1986). The synopsis record card: a stepping stone to the computer. *Journal of the Royal College of General Practitioners*, **36**, 564–6.
12. Preece, J. (1990). *The use of computers in general practice*, 2nd. edn. Churchill Livingstone, London.
13. Aylett, M. (1985). Computerised repeat prescriptions: simple system. *British Medical Journal*, **290**, 1115–6.
14. Donald, J. B. (1989). Prescribing costs when computers are used to issue all prescriptions. *British Medical Journal*, **299**, 28–30.
15. Telling, J. P., Davies, K. R., Difford, F., Fornear, J. E., and Reading, C. A. (1984). Developing a practice formulary as a by-product of computer controlled repeat prescribing. *British Medical Journal*, **288**, 1730–2.
16. Mills, K. A., Steele, K., and Irwin, W. G. (1988). A computerized audit of non-steroidal anti-inflammatory drug prescribing in general practice. *Family Practice*, **5**, 40–5.
17. Melville, A. W. T. (1989). Patient access to general practice medical records. *Health Bulletin*, **47**, 5–8.

11. The efficient consulting-room

INTRODUCTION

It is probably true that a general practitioner spends more time in his consulting-room than he does in almost any other room during the whole of his life. Therefore, he must feel at home and comfortable there, and it may well be allowed to reflect some of his characteristics (the more acceptable ones that is!) Personal items such as favourite paintings, flowers, statuary, attractive vases, plants, and photographs of members of his own family should identify the room as his own. Where a room has to be shared, it is possible with thought to interchange the 'personal items' depending on who is actually in it. But in an ideal world general practitioners should have their own consulting-room, and this is increasingly important as the time spent outside the surgery decreases (see Chapter 3). Even when not consulting, the room will serve as an office and study.

Having said all that, however, the room should also be efficient, and it is the aim of this chapter to illustrate that comfort and ambience do not preclude this.

PATIENT FLOW

There should be a steady flow of patients from the main waiting-room, ideally to a small sub-waiting-area just outside the doctor's door. It is always better if one or two people are waiting there: the patient who enters the doctor's room thinking she is the only person to be seen that morning, sometimes tries to take the whole of it!

Summoning the patient from outside the consulting-room can be done by means of 'traffic lights—'come in', 'wait', 'engaged'—controlled from the doctor's desk. This avoids spending time and effort ushering patients in and out. Patients rapidly learn the system that their doctor uses, and if it is simple and efficient they accept it.

The records and the computer screen should be immediately available to the doctor on his desk and the prescription printer near the patient's chair, so that she can take the prescription as soon as it emerges (see Chapter 10).

The doctor's desk should be so sited that he can watch the patients enter the room; first, to catch their overall demeanour, secondly to study their movements, and thirdly, perhaps importantly at a time of increasing aggression, can be aware of any belligerent attitude in the patient.[1-3]

Consultation across the corner of a table or desk seems to be extremely popular.[4,5] Increasingly the desk is becoming less significant and less of a barrier in the room, and the unimpeded face-to-face position of doctor and patient of greater importance. I find that by consulting across the right-hand corner of a table, which I have done for about twenty years, I can have my 'office' facilities to my left hand—the telephone, computer screen, records, and so on—and with my right hand, can reach the patient. Access is aided by having a chair with efficient castors, that runs easily to and fro across the carpet. Much thought should be given by doctors to the sort of chair they wish to sit in—it is the chair in their life which they will spend the longest time in.[6] Mine has arms, is well padded and comfortable, tips back, swivels, and runs easily. A reclining chair is important in the busily efficient practice, since a patient's desire to talk can be encouraged by that sense of leisureliness induced by the doctor leaning back in a relaxed attitude. In a large proportion of consultations no examination is indicated. In a further large group the examination couch is not used, and chair-to-chair access for limited examination is all that is necessary. I can take the pulse, check ankles for oedema, examine limbs, look in throats, and listen to hearts without actually leaving my chair. To palpate cervical glands, examine neck-movements, listen to the lung bases, and feel the sites of various injuries and aches and pains, I have to stand up and sometimes walk round the patient's chair; similarly to look in ears. But the classical examinations of efficient general practice can be geographically circumscribed affairs.

The patient too needs a comfortable chair and the ability to rest an arm on the desk, just as the doctor does. Near to the patient's hand should be a box of tissues, and these will also be available to the doctor. The patient's chair should be easy to get in and out of. There should also be another one for relatives, and a third one at the other side of the room, if yet another person comes in. Small children accompanying adults need to be accommodated and entertained within the efficient consulting-room; the presence of toys, a toy-box, or a doll's house to play with under the consulting-room couch or in some corner, frequently takes the pressure off parents trying to describe their problem.[7]

There should be easy access from both patient's and doctor's chair to the examination couch, which in the efficient practice should be in the consulting-room. The couch should have curtains which can be drawn round it so that the patient can dress and undress in privacy. With the well-known doctor and well-known patient this is frequently unnecessary, but nevertheless it is good that the patient should have the option of privacy. There should be hooks to hang clothes on both by the couch and by the chair. Whilst a patient is dressing and undressing the doctor can do other things—write notes, enter computer data, complete pathology forms and so on.

There should be a very convenient hand-basin for both doctor and patient to use after the examination and individual towels for each. In my room, I provide two glass tumblers, one each for patient and doctor, since an occasional sip of water is appreciated by both. I used to have a prominent supply of my favourite analgesic tablets (on the 'blacklist' of course), but found that I used these only for myself and never for patients. They were also raided by the receptionists; I now hide them.

CLINICAL EQUIPMENT

There are two examination sites in the consulting-room, and there should be a supply of equipment at each of them; this means having two of virtually everything in the consulting-room.

Available at the chair/desk site I have several duckets on the wall at my right hand containing blood-pressure machine, tendom hammer complete with brush and pricker in the handle, pen-torch, tape-measure, magnifying glass, blunt-ended scissors, auriscope with several speculums, mini-swabs for cleaning them, ophthalmoscope, tongue depressors, middle-C tuning fork, height/weight calculator, FEV gadgets for adults and children, cotton wool, thermometers—normal and low registering, and a stethoscope. In addition there are supplies of prescription pads, certificates of various types, and a 'tick-off' form for patients to use for making other appointments—vascular clinic, well-man clinic, minor ops, and so on. All these items are accommodated in a 9-ducket open-fronted piece of shelving no larger than three feet by three feet. Every one of them can be reached and used with only a small movement of the chair on its castors. Some doctors use a nearby trolley and others the old-fashioned, but very functional, multi-drawered roll-top desk. The overriding principle is that the items are immediately available, always in good working order (the efficient receptionist should see to that once a week), and accessible without leaving the chair.[8]

Two larger items are available very close to the patient's chair. One is a wall-mounted height measure, used infrequently since most people know their height, and a pair of small bathroom scales which can be kicked under the table or chair when not in use. There is no doubt that my weighing of patients increased enormously—and certainly gave both patient and myself several surprises—when scales were available literally next to the patient's feet.

All the above instruments (except scales and height measure) are replicated on the shelf over the examination couch. The blood-pressure machine is in fact fixed to the wall to save space. One addition on the shelf is a foetal stethoscope.

By having examination instruments available both at the couch and at the chair there is no carrying from one to the other nor, even worse, leaving items at the couch and having them unavailable for the next patient at the chair.

Next to, or under, the couch there are shelves or drawers containing trays for various examinations. For example, there should be a gynae tray which would include cervical cytology equipment and high-vaginal swabs, a throat tray for swabs, and also an eye tray (eye spud and needle, drops, cotton buds, and so on). These will be used relatively infrequently but to have them instantly available is vital. I recently 'designed' a proctoscope tray, and find that the number of rectums I have actually inspected has arisen merely because the tray is there. Provision of equipment encourages thorough examination and results in more accurate diagnosis.

The walls of the consulting-room can be useful for 'charts'. In a 'clinical corner' in my room I have an Oxford Growth Screening wall-chart for children aged 2 to 9 years—an immediate reassurance to anxious parents that their children are growing appropriately. To supplement this I have a supply of height/weight charts in a cupboard in another corner of the room, as well as height/weight charts for older age-groups. To some extent this awaits body-mass indices from age/height/weight calculations becoming automatically available on the patient's computer screen.

On the wall above the couch I have a Snellen's test type card which can be illuminated by an appropriately sited angle-poise lamp. I can use the lamp also for taking swabs from vagina, throat, and so on. Opposite the Snellen's card is a mark on the carpet at exactly three metres so that a patient's eyes can be tested at the correct distance.

Also on the wall, I have an obstetric calculator for working out expected dates of delivery, a peak expiratory flow calculator giving norms for PEF by age, height, and sex, and also several coloured anatomy charts showing simple pictures of a hiatus hernia, peptic ulcer, duodenal and gastric ulcerations, and simple diagrams of the coronary arteries showing how angina is caused and what happens in a myocardial infarction. These charts are sufficiently large that they can be seen across the consulting-room from the patient's and doctor's chair, and I use a small spotlight indicator to illustrate on the chart what I am talking about. Finally I have an anatomical chart of the female genito-urinary tract which is useful for demonstrating intra-uterine contraceptive devices, pelvic inflammatory disease, cervical smear, and so on. Such visual aids facilitate not only an efficient consultation but also a thorough one. Everything is to hand or to eye.

In a cupboard in the room near the doctor's chair, are a series of some twenty to thirty folders in different colours. They are all named and in alphabetical order. They contain 'hand-outs' for the patients on various topics, from exercises for various muscular groups—back, neck, quadriceps, pelvic-floor, and so on—to treating a verruca with formalin solution, general advice about acne, and mobilization after a myocardial infarction. After a few weeks, I could no longer remember exactly what I had put into the folders in the cupboard, so on my desk I have an index of them; at a glance I can recall which are there, and the different-coloured files make identification easy.

Also in the cupboard, which is divided into various cubby-holes, is an asthma section. In it are samples of all my customarily prescribed asthma equipment: there is a pressurized inhaler with placebo canister for demonstration purposes, rotahaler with placebo capsules, nebuhaler, and so on. These are items from the practice minicopoeia plus some alternatives for complicated patients (see Chapter 6).

CLINICAL DATA READY TO HAND

Immediate availability of clinical data saves an enormous amount of time, effort, and racking of brains. It requires only a small amount of forethought to collect a list of commonly needed data at consultations over a period of several months. Once assembled, it can be placed in the table or desk drawer, or in a cubby-hole at arm's length. Here are some of mine:

Prescribing data

(1) Practice 'minicopoeia';

(2) *The National Formulary*;

(3) MIMS.

(Most patients like to see doctors looking things up. To them it ensures accuracy and demonstrates concern.)

The National Formulary contains various important sections under 'guidance on prescribing'. Amongst those I use most frequently are 'prescribing in pregnancy' and 'prescribing during breastfeeding'. There is also a useful appendix on drug interactions, but its length and detail make it somewhat daunting. Nevertheless, for the occasional patient with complicated therapy it can be of great value. For less-difficult problems, I use a splendid 'medisc' which was the result of much research and was produced by 'Excerpta Medica Services Inc. 1976'. In disc-form are the interactions of all the common drugs with each other and also with alcohol.

One of the drug firms also produces an easy-to-use check-list on 'A Guide to Drugs in Breast Milk'—easier to use than *The National Formulary*.

Drug groups and which to choose

Available from drug firms are lists of various types of drug. For example, non-steroidal anti-inflammatory drugs are listed according to type, so that when changing from one to the other doctors can be sure that they are actually changing the pharmacology, that is switching from a propionic-acid derivative to an acetic-acid derivative rather than merely from one propionic acid to another. Favourite NSAIDs, those in the 'minicopoeia', or the cheaper ones, can be underlined. The various anti-depressants can be divided into three groups—sedative, neutral, and stimulant—and again appropriate choices and switches made. The oral contraceptives are another jungle which the minicopoeia can help; side-effects and the appropriate alternatives are available in disc-form.

Laboratory tests

Immediate access to lists of the normal levels for haematology, biochemistry, and so on, in an easily accessible drawer in a desk is valuable. Local hospitals sometimes produce their own 'in-house' list of normals and obviously these are the ones that should be available.

Prescriptions

The desktop computer and printer within the consulting-room have revolutionized acute prescribing (see Chapter 4). For those still awaiting this change, however, prescription headings—name, age, address—should always have been completed by receptionists and be available with the patient's record. When patients request repeat prescriptions during the consultation, the doctor should direct the patient to make the request from the receptionist who, using the computer, will be able to ensure its accuracy. If patients get into the habit of requesting repeat prescriptions via the doctor they will never learn to use the receptionists appropriately.

OFFICE 'AIDS' READY TO HAND

Usually on the desk, but certainly available within arm's length, should be a rack of updated haematology, pathology, and X-ray forms, and the like, along with all appropriate stationery. Doctors should not fill in these forms apart from the clinical notes on them. The names, addresses, ages, and other details should be completed by clerical staff. In my practice this is done by clipping the forms on to the front of the record folder, which then goes to reception to be completed. From there they are made available to the nurses taking the tests (blood, and so on) when the patient presents.

Also at arm's length should be some sort of 'intercom system'—we use a British Telecom telephone system but there are many others—so that there is immediate access to members of the team. Accordingly, receptionists can be asked for extra records of family members, the secretary given an urgent letter via telephone shorthand, a partner invited to give a second opinion, or a trainee summoned to see an interesting problem. Telephones can be 'programmed' to give automatic lines to frequently used numbers such as local hospitals, home, and so on, but for the most part receptionists should be used to getting appropriate people on the line, so long as the doctor is immediately available to take the call.

THE EFFICIENT CONSULTING-ROOM FROM THE PATIENT'S POINT OF VIEW

Patients are reassured if the doctor they consult seems well-organized, with all his instruments conveniently to hand and information and 'handouts' readily available. Fumbling and disorganization, although at times endearing and charming, can sometimes be associated with similar attitudes to clinical knowledge! Patients like to be able to lean on the desk and relax in a pleasant chair. They enjoy a positioning of furniture which establishes rapport and ambience as well as being efficient. They respect the thoughtfulness of the provision of tissues, hand-washing facilities, a drink of water—and even an occasional analgesic from the secret cupboard.

REFERENCES

1. D'Urso, P. and Hobbs, R. (1989). Aggression and the general practitioner. *British Medical Journal*, **298**, 97–8.
2. Harris, A. (1989). Violence in general practice. *British Medical Journal*, **298**, 63–4.
3. Breakwell, G. M. (1989). *Facing physical violence*. Routledge, London.
4. Cammock, R. (1981). *Primary health care buildings*. Architectural Press, London.
5. Cox, A. and Groves, P. (1981). *Design for health care*. Butterworths, London.
6. Edwards, K. (1978). The environment in practice. *Practitioner*, **221**, 465–9.
7. Jolleys, J. V. (1987). How to present an attractive shop front. *Practitioner*, **35**, 1335–7.
8. Drury, M. and Collin, M. (1986). *The medical secretary's and receptionist's handbook*, 5th edn. Bailliere, London.

12. Working fast

SHORT, SHARP SURGERIES

Like most of the animal kingdom, doctors are brighter and quicker earlier in the day than they are towards the end of it. Hence starting work at 8.30 a.m. with an early-morning surgery can give a momentum to the day which will serve the doctor in good stead when caring for large numbers of patients. Indeed, some practices now have a surgery at 8.00 a.m., which provides an opportunity for working patients to attend *en route* for work, and is also available for those coming off night-shift. Research has repeatedly shown that a doctor's energy and intellect flags towards the end of long consulting sessions; the consultations tend to become longer but simultaneously less effective.[1,2] Hence it is more efficient if surgery sessions are never longer than an hour and a half, and are interspersed by team meetings, coffee breaks, teaching, administration, organizational sessions, and home visits. Many doctors now have surgeries between 8.30 and 10.00 a.m., 11.30 and 12.30 p.m., 2.00 and 3.30 p.m., and 4.00 and 5.30 p.m. If a doctor runs late in such an appointment system, the overrunning time is reduced: there is only half the 'overrunning' time in an hour-and-a-half session than there is in a three-hour session. Although the numbers of patients attending each of these sessions may well be only between ten and fifteen, it is advisable to book the early part of the session at shorter intervals and space later patients at longer ones. Thus patients are never 'alone', and therefore do not assume that the doctor is 'not busy' and decide to expand on multiple problems which might otherwise be more circumscribed. I double-book my attendances between 8.30 and 8.45 a.m.; if some of these early bookings are cancelled, or arrive late, I do not find myself with no-one to see when I am in the best state of mind to be working hard.

Ideally, patients should wait immediately outside the doctor's sound-proofed room, and there should be an even flow of them to this sub-waiting area. The days when the doctor walked through to the waiting-room and shouted: 'Next!' have gone. Some patients can be directed by receptionists to spare consulting or examination rooms, if the doctor has forewarned the receptionist that a comprehensive examination will be necessary. A quick look through the record envelopes at the beginning of a session can sometimes indicate which patients these will be: the elderly, for example, are often candidates.

Careful study of the practice geography can facilitate short, sharp visiting sessions to well-circumscribed areas. But home visits are decreasing and becoming a much smaller component of the doctor's day (see Chapter 3). I have found that if only a short time is allocated for visits, the time actually spent is reduced—it seems that visits expand to fill the visiting-time provided!

THE MERITS OF THE QUICK CONSULTATION

The virtues of the long consultation are well known—it is warm and comforting, it is usually thorough, it reveals hidden problems, it is associated with more comprehensive examination, it is thought to be associated with fewer prescriptions and fewer antibiotics, and it elicits high patient satisfaction; but the quick consultation too has merits and obviously in this book these will be emphasized.[3-5] It is important to remember that it is facilitated by having a personal list where multiple consultations over many years by known doctor and known patient lead to efficiency in the time used (Chapter 8). If this previous care has been clearly recorded by the doctor, either in writing or on the computer, then he can rapidly refer to earlier notes when appropriate (see Chapter 10).

The average consultation in the United Kingdom is somewhere between six and seven minutes; this has been substantiated in many studies.[6,7] Therefore if some consultations are as long as ten or twenty minutes, and all doctors will have experience of these, this must mean that to produce an average of six or seven there must be consultations of three, four, or five minutes. In my own practice I timed all my consultations for a period of six months. The data which emerged are probably reasonably representative of many doctors who try to work efficiently and fairly quickly. My average overall consultation time was 6.1 minutes. However, major new diagnoses resulted in an average consultation time of 13 minutes; follow-up of major diagnoses an average of 7 minutes; minor new illnesses, follow-up of minor illnesses, and repeat episodes of the same minor illness averaged about 5 minutes. Hence the clinical conditions themselves—perhaps obviously—largely dictated the length of the consultation. In other studies this simple fact has not been sufficiently highlighted. Because of the large number of consultations about minor conditions, 34 per cent of my overall consultations took less than 4 minutes. Put simply, 'little' conditions require little time. The patient's age made a significant difference; those who were over 13 years old averaged 6–7 minutes; children under 13 averaged 4¾ minutes, and 58 per cent of their consultations took less than 4 minutes. Patently it is children—happily the vast majority with only minor illness—that can be seen quickly. Sometimes two or three children in the same family will be brought to the same consultation, will have the same diagnosis, and will need identical therapy; their average consultation time will be very short indeed.

It is important that minor illnesses are not aggrandized.[8] If they are, then despite all manner of health education, patients will conclude that it is appropriate to consult for such conditions on subsequent occasions. Likewise, if a consultation is a rerun of a former trivial problem—and here good records are vital—then the rerun itself should be speedy. Many people, and particularly young adults, do not quite know the function of the doctor and when they should consult. If minor illnesses are trivialized they rapidly become aware that attendances for them are probably inappropriate. There is not a major psycho-social problem lurking within every consultation for minor illness. The good doctor knows when it is there, and for the rest he 'trivializes the trivial'.

When, occasionally, a long consultation does take place it is probably important to write in the notes 'long chat', or words to that effect, to serve as a reminder to the doctor that the patient has had a very long consultation about that particular problem. Hence he does not repeat this exercise every time.

By working quickly with short consultation-times doctors can certainly increase the number of patients on their list. Just as importantly, if many short consultations take place for minor conditions, this does allow more time for the serious problems.

WORKING FAST FROM THE PATIENT'S POINT OF VIEW

Patients prefer their doctor to be fresh and bright when they consult him, so attendances early in the day are more rewarding. They prefer the multiple consultation times provided in three or four sessions throughout the day, since these are more likely to fit in with work, family, social, or other commitments. Short surgery sessions reduce overrunning time, and this is appreciated by patients. Not having to wait is equated with efficiency, and efficiency they associate with accuracy and expertise. Patients do not object to quick consultations so long as the doctor gets to the root of the problem and the management is effective. They too have busy lives and have better things to do with their time than spending half an hour discussing the far end of their varicose veins.

In my patient-satisfaction survey several questions were asked about whether patients felt hurried, or not examined sufficiently, or that they could discuss more than one problem at a time, and so on.[9] Against a background of a five- to six-minute average consultation, 90 per cent of those questioned felt that they were able to tell the doctor all they wanted to about their health. The doctor always or often gave them sufficient time and 'did not hurry them', and he virtually always explained things fully and answered all their questions. Very similar high satisfaction was expressed about the thoroughness of the examination and the carrying out of tests. It would seem that in the five- to six-minute consultation a great deal can be achieved. Professor Anthony Clare, when observing many consultations in general practice through a two-way mirror was impressed by the fact that there 'never seemed to be any rush'; this was against a background of consultations lasting only five or six minutes.[10]

All in all, speed does not preclude a high level of patient satisfaction; because of it a much larger number of patients can be seen.

REFERENCES

1. Eimerl, T. S. and Pearson, R. J. C. (1966). Working-time in general practice. How general practitioners use their time. *British Medical Journal*, **2**, 1549–54.
2. Williams, W. D. (1970). *A study of general practitioners' workload in South Wales 1965–1966*. Report from general practice. RCGP, London.
3. Morrell, D. C., Evans, M. E., Morris, R. W. and Roland, M. D. (1988). The 'five minute' consultation: effect of time constraints on clinical content and patient satisfaction. *British Medical Journal*, **292**, 870–73.
4. Howie, J. G. R., Porter, A. M. D., and Forbes, J. F. (1989). Quality and the use of time in general practice: widening the discussion. *British Medical Journal*, **298**, 1008–10.
5. Cartwright, A. and Anderson, R. (1981). *General practice revisited*. Tavistock, London.
6. Buchan, I. C. and Richardson, I. M. (1973). *Time study of consultations in general practice*. Scottish Home and Health Department, Edinburgh.
7. Fry, J. (edn.) (1979). *Trends in general practice 1979*. BMJ, London.
8. Marsh, G. N. (1977). 'Curing' minor illness in general practice. *British Medical Journal*, **2**, 1267–9.
9. Marsh, G. N. and Kaim-Caudle, P. (1976). *Team care in general practice*. Croom Helm, London.
10. Clare, A. Personal Communication, 1982.

13. Using the telephone

INTRODUCTION

There is only occasional mention of the use of the telephone in literature from general practice in the United Kingdom.[1-3] Perhaps this is not surprising in a country where home visiting is still considered sacrosanct by both patients and doctors. Nevertheless, as home visiting is reducing (see Chapter 3), telephone communication is becoming more important. In countries such as Canada and the USA, where there is little or no home visiting, there have been many studies of the effectiveness of telephone consultations.[4-8] Overall, the results have been encouraging. The telephone is a major means of communication and every efficient practice should consider its use. Analyses of consultations in general practice show that in a large proportion of them the patient is not examined.[9] Hence the history is all important, and this can be taken over the telephone. Also of supreme importance are the patients' comprehensive records open in front of the doctor, with earlier examinations and past diagnoses and therapies clearly noted (see Chapter 10).[10]

It is important to remember that the telephone is a two-way machine. Whereas traditionally patients rang their doctor, now doctors in efficient practices are ringing their patients.

THE ROUTINE PRACTICE TELEPHONE SYSTEM

Telephones have become much more sophisticated in the last ten or fifteen years, as part of the technological revolution. This book is not the place to describe the various systems; suffice to say that British Telecom, as well as private telephone firms, are only too happy to monitor and assess the needs of the practice and make appropriate recommendations. The remainder of this chapter will describe how important the telephone is, but there is no doubt that to have the most sophisticated and up-to-date machinery available is vital. Most importantly, there must be sufficient telephone lines so that patients can get through with ease and doctors and staff are able to ring out from the premises without having to wait for lines to clear. Plenty of lines require plenty of people to answer them. In large practices with busy common-rooms frequently thronged with people, it may well be necessary to have two, three, or more telephones in the same room. In our own practice, a long table down the centre of the common-room has three telephones on it. Occasionally at coffee and tea time all three phones can be in use (see Chapter 2). The telephonist must know which telephone particular team members sit beside.

Patients often form their first impression of the practice from the type of reception they get when they telephone the surgery. An immediate answer suggests efficiency. A calmly sympathetic voice, patently welcoming the call and expressing interest, is ideal. Receptionists are not necessarily the most appropriate people to answer the telephone, since with a comprehensive team the proportion of calls merely to make appointments has fallen considerably. Frequently patients or other callers are wishing to speak to any member of the team, including the increasingly large number of administrative staff. Hence an increasing need for a telephonist. By using a small 'exchange' the telephonist can ensure a rapid response to ascertain the type of call and then direct it to the appropriate person. Callers can be told whether a short wait will be necessary, and reassured from time to time if the wait becomes longer than was at first anticipated. Within the practice it is important that, when a phone rings and someone is available to answer it, it should not ring more than twice before it is picked up: the 'two-ring' rule. Thus the person ringing, telephonist or other member of staff, will know rapidly whether there is someone there or not.

There should be almost no interruptions of doctors' and nurses' consulting sessions. Where there has to be, the 'two-ring rule' applies. However, such calls should be for dire emergencies, for other in-calling doctors and nurses who cannot ring back, and for the doctors' spouse! The great majority of people wishing to speak to a doctor or nurse will be told when to ring or, alternatively and increasingly, the doctor or nurse will return the call (see later).

The duty doctor, available for emergencies, must make the telephonist aware of where he is throughout the working day. If he leaves the building the telephonist should be told, so that she can contact him by whatever system the practice uses ('bleep', car phone, and so on). In the evening and at night, there must be an immediate system of access via a 'bleep' or other paging system. It is helpful if there is one telephone-number to the practice which is known only to the team members; when they are out in the community and wish to make contact they can use this infrequently used line knowing that it will seldom be 'engaged'. This is particularly vital for midwives or nurses who may well be involved in sudden emergency situations.

On the whole, clinical staff should not initiate calls themselves; this should be part of the expertise of receptionists. It is essential, however, that the clinical staff-member requesting the call must be immediately available to take it. So, having asked a clerk to get someone on the telephone, the doctor or nurse must sit in their room and not use their telephone until the call has been put through, or the non-availability of the person called has been ascertained.

Admitting patients to hospital should be almost entirely the work of the reception staff. The receptionist, having been given the details of the case from the doctor, can then ring the appropriate bed bureau, ward, or hospital doctor concerned, describe the problem, and arrange the admission. If necessary, she can put the hospital doctor through to the practice doctor for further discussion. By the same token, a great deal of telephone work can now be done between doctors' secretaries, particularly with reference to organizing early appointments, looking for delayed hospital reports and investigations, arranging urgent tests, and so on.

THE 'TELEPHONE HALF-HOUR'

In the efficient practice there will be a time in the doctor's day (often this is convenient immediately after the team meeting), when he is available to receive incoming telephone calls and also has time to make outgoing ones. Indeed, not only doctors require this 'telephone half-hour', but so probably do other members of the team—health-visitors, nurses, midwives, and the rest. This period is set aside for people who have already rung when the doctor or nurse was consulting or busy, and they have been told to ring back. Alternatively telephone numbers can be taken—this happens increasingly—and the doctor rings them. The problem with asking patients to ring back is that this produces a jam of incoming calls, and all the practice lines become engaged. In terms of staff time, as well as practice efficiency, it is probably worth paying for the expense of the calls. By and large, clinical members of the team retreat to their rooms for their 'telephone half-hour'. If the half-hour can be staggered, this causes less strain on the system.

TELEPHONE CONSULTATIONS INSTEAD OF FACE-TO-FACE CONSULTATION

The most important feature in the telephone consultation is that the doctor should have the patient's record in front of him. If personal lists operate, then this naturally aids the consultation: patient and doctor know each other well and have consulted over many illnesses across the years, and the records are readily scrutinized.

The consultation should always be recorded when done on the telephone as part of the continuum of care, and it is useful when face-to-face consultation ultimately takes place. It is also important from the medico-legal viewpoint. The following are fairly random examples of recent telephone consultations done in my own practice which illustrate their value and breadth:

1. A man with an exacerbation of gout who is not on Allopurinol and for whom I prescribed high-dose Indomethacin with instructions to consult later.

2. A five-month old baby with a hot, flushed arm around an injection site for triple antigen carried out the day before. I explained that this was a not-uncommon local-sensitivity reaction, and advised cold Calamine lotion and Paracetamol if required.

3. A woman with post-herpetic neuralgia three weeks after a zoster rash. Previously prescribed analgesics were proving ineffective, and I increased the strength of them from Paracetamol to Co-dydramol.

4. An exacerbation of previously diagnosed recurrent headache in a woman under considerable stress. A previous good response to Prochlorperazine. I prescribed this again.

5. Adjusting medication for a severely epileptic child.

6. A woman of 22 whom I had seen the day before with an upper-respiratory-tract infection and swollen throat and prescribed Paracetamol. Now with a Scarlatiniform rash and with known Scarlatina in one of her children. I prescribed Penicillin (perhaps I should have done this the day before!)

7. An 80-year-old depressive female not responding particularly well to one Phenelzine tablet a day—she had in the past taken two with better effect. I advised her to increase the dose and consult later.

8. Patient with chronic heart-failure requiring increase in diuretic because of slight worsening of oedema of feet. Arranged nurse to visit for follow-up and biochemistry.

9. Advising a distraught teenager what to do about her delayed period, possibly an unwanted pregnancy. Gave advice about urine collection for pregnancy test and the need for consultation twenty-four hours after that.

10. Advising a patient whose 'back has gone again'. Customary bed-rest and analgesics and programme of mobility. Had several previous episodes.

11. A male of 38 with an exacerbation of his iritis. Left prescription for steroid drops and advised to reconsult in a few days if not settling.

12. Prescription for another episode of tonsillitis in a child of 6 awaiting tonsillectomy. Mother reports yellow spots on tonsils and temperature for three days. Left prescription for Penicillin V.

13. Child of 5 with recurrence of earache associated with respiratory infection. Earache has lasted on and off for twenty-four hours with fever. Left prescription for Penicillin V and instructions to follow-up in a few days at the surgery.

14. A woman of 22 with a repeat episode of acute cystitis. Left prescription for short course of Trimethoprim with instructions to have urine culture if symptoms not totally resolved at end of the course.

15. Man with severe cough and painful ribs seen the previous day, but X-ray not arranged on that occasion. Left form for X-ray of ribs and to reconsult later.

16. Advice to sister at nursing-home about interval changes of care necessary between routine weekly visits to the nursing-home. (Routine weekly visits are done because I have thirty-five patients there.)

It is also possible to give the results of investigations and tests on the telephone and there seems little reason why the doctor should not call patients at home and give them results. All this saves consultations, many of which now end with the comment 'I will ring you if anything turns up'; patients can assume that no news is good news.

Perhaps the most frequent way for patients to receive results in my own practice is by being told to ask the receptionist for them. Blood lipids, ESRs in rheumatic disease, negative chest X-rays, follow-up urine cultures, and full blood-counts to show improvement on haematinics are the sort of laboratory reports that can be paraphrased in simple English by the doctor, and the receptionist can relay this message to the patient. The major problem is remembering which patients have been told to use this system; putting 'LM' (Leave Message) on the relevant laboratory-investigation form reminds me that this patient is going to enquire and that I must write appropriately on the form when the result comes back from the laboratory. The clinical problem must be recorded on the request form in enough detail to enable the doctor to leave his message without the need for consulting the record again. There are potentially all sorts of 'aids' that can be used to make sure the system runs smoothly, but the underlying principle is that receptionists can, and should be trained to, give messages to patients regarding the results of tests and progress they are making. Even hospitals—never places at the forefront of operational efficiency— are now writing or telephoning patients to save out-patient attendances.

At follow-up attendances at the surgery patients frequently do not need to be re-examined; only a history of their progress needs to be elicited. It seems to me that again not enough use is made of the telephone; perhaps increasingly a consultation should end with 'if you don't get better within [giving however long the condition should take] then give me a ring. My telephone half-hour is 10.30 to 11 a.m. except on Tuesdays.' Doctors generate a lot of their own consultative work by asking patients to come back to see them; they could save the patients and the practice staff a lot of trouble and time by getting the patient to use the phone.

In the same way, the telephone can be used instead of carrying out follow-up home visits; this has already been emphasized (see Chapter 3). All repeat visits should be scrutinized to see which of them can be done on the phone—possibly most of them.

OUT-OF-HOURS TELEPHONE WORK

When on duty, the doctor should find himself sitting in a comfortable armchair, the book in which he records evening and night telephone consultations next to his right hand, and a mobile telephone at his left.[11] Thus 'armed', it should be his aim to give advice about 'urgent medical emergencies' (to quote our surgery tape) without leaving his chair. When the patient rings then the doctor always speaks. As a matter of principle no patient will be refused a visit, but after taking an appropriate history advice should be proffered. One golden rule is that, once advice has been given on the telephone but the patient or relative ring again expressing further concern, then a visit should be made. In my own study of telephone usage in out-of-hours work, 65 per cent of telephone calls between 6 p.m. and 8 a.m., and Saturday afternoons and Sundays, were responded to on the telephone. My less-experienced partner did about 50 per cent, giving us an overall average of a 59 per cent telephone response. This percentage was the same even for so-called 'out of bed' calls received between 11 p.m. and 8 a.m., and we had the second-lowest reported night-call rate in the United Kingdom. Even with the trebling of the night-call fee from £15 to £45, it is unlikely that we will change our system—our beds are comfortable! Also, 36 per cent of the telephone calls concerned patients who were already on treatment for acute or chronic conditions, that is, not for new problems. Thus, in 36 per cent of cases the diagnosis had been made, the therapy was already established, and all that was required was some modification of management because of a new development. Of the new problems on the telephone, a large proportion were for upper-respiratory-tract infections and gastro-intestinal disturbances, especially diarrhoea. Our results showed that it was easier to give telephone advice for children than for the elderly, in whom the pathology was more serious.

The 'armchair routine', therefore, is to take a history, ideally from the patient herself. Not infrequently relatives ring up about a patient who is perfectly able to speak on the phone herself. The known doctor and the known patient conversing together immediately generates a rapport which is impossible via a third party. From their discussions, the problem can be assessed and one of four courses of action can follow:

(1) an immediate and urgent visit;

(2) a visit, but later, when other visits may have accumulated;

(3) an attendance at surgery at an appropriate time (35 per cent of telephone calls advised to come to the surgery did not come at all: patently the telephone advice was all that was necessary);

(4) telephone advice, with the strict instruction that if the problem does not ameliorate as a result then the patient or relative must ring back. A second telephone call is virtually always responded to by a visit.

USING THE TELEPHONE FROM THE PATIENT'S POINT OF VIEW

Patients greatly appreciate a doctor who will speak to them on the telephone; it is far less bother than coming to the surgery. They welcome being able to discuss 'a small point' or indulge in 'a quick query'. Indeed, they often feel that the paraphernalia of making an appointment, getting ready, attending the surgery, and being seen is really just 'not worth it'. For the doctor to return a call is looked upon as friendly and considerate— and so, I suppose, it is. The steadying voice in the evening about anxieties concerning a hot child, a tummy-ache, or a diarrhoea is very welcome.

REFERENCES

1. Weingarten, M. A. (1982). Telephone consultations with patients: a brief study and review of the literature. *Journal of the Royal College of General Practitioners*, **32**, 766–70.
2. McCarthy, M. and Bollam, M. (1990). Telephone advice for out of hours calls in general practice. *British Journal of General Practice*, **40**, 19–21.

3. Allsop, J. and May, A. (1985). *Telephone access to GPs in the UK: a study of London*. King Edward's Hospital Fund, London.
4. Westbury, R. C. (1974). The electric speaking practice: a telephone workload study. *Canadian Family Physician*, **20 (2)**, 69–76.
5. Perrin, E. C. and Goodman, H. C. (1978). Telephone management of acute paediatric illness. *New England Journal of Medicine*, **298**, 130–5.
6. Radeck, S. E., Neville, R. E. and Girard, R. A. (1989). Telephone patient management by primary care physicians. *Medical Care*, **27**, 817–22.
7. Daugird, A. J. (1988). Patient telephone call documentation: quality implications and an attempted intervention. *Journal of Family Practice*, **27**, 420–1.
8. Curtis, P. and Evens, S. (1989). Doctor–patient communication on the telephone. *Canadian Family Physician*, **35**, 123–8.
9. Marsh, G. N., Wallace, R. B., and Whewell, J. (1976). Anglo-American contrasts in general practice. *British Medical Journal*, **1**, 1321–5.
10. Marsh, G. N. and Thornham, J. R. (1980). Changing to A4 folders and updating records in a 'busy' general practice. *British Medical Journal*, **281**, 215–17.
11. Marsh, G. N., Horne, R. A. and Channing, D. M. (1987). A study of telephone advice in managing out-of-hours calls. *Journal of the Royal College of General Practitioners*, **37**, 301–4.

14. Involving patients

Faced with a doctor's 'efficient style', patients automatically become involved in 'efficiency'. In particular, doctors who run personal lists know that their patients get to know the way they work and how to comply best to get the best out of the system (see Chapter 8).[1,2] They are well aware, probably from many many consultations, that he expects them to come to the point of their problem fairly promptly, and if it is thought to be helpful he encourages them to bring lists of problems, symptoms, and so on so that these can be readily discussed. Patients know when the doctor is busy, first from the length of time they may have had to wait for a non-urgent appointment, and secondly from having to wait beyond their appointment time until they are actually seen. Frequently the doctor's demeanour shows how busy he is and the need for a neatly circumscribed consultation. Obviously the confused patient with a major problem will be unable to concur with any of the above, and will need, and must receive, a lot of time; but for the most part patients can, and will, comply.

This chapter, however, is more particularly about the tangible aids to efficiency that patients can expect to receive in modern practice. Just as when people sign on with a building society, insurance company, or even a bank, such institutions make considerable efforts to apprise their new members of their aims, and the quality and extent of the services offered, so too can the doctor and his practice hand out leaflets, brochures, and so on to familiarize patients more quickly with what the practice has to offer. This has become more necessary as the scope and facilities of practices have increased—well evidenced by the previous chapters in this book. The time when a new patient registering with a general practitioner was lucky to receive a card with the telephone-numbers and surgery times, or even nothing more than a curt nod from a busy receptionist, have gone. The major 'document' is now the 'practice brochure', and its involvement in the efficient working of the practice will be highlighted first in this chapter.

PRACTICE BROCHURE

Practice brochures have become extremely common, especially since the introduction of the 'new contract'.[3-5] But they were gradually increasing before that, ever since the first one emanating from my own practice was described in the British Medical Journal in 1980. Indeed, since the 'new contract', the family-health services authorities are making them actually mandatory. Many practices are starting to use them not just for their own patients, but also as a form of advertising for people who live in the area but who are not patients of the practice. The relaxation of rules on advertising has given a considerable fillip to the production of practice brochures.[6]

The first edition of our brochure—it is now in its third—was a relatively humble, twenty-two-page booklet with simple cartoons and a somewhat folksy style. The paper written around its research was entitled 'The practice brochure—a patient's guide to team care', and this title emphasized its considerable orientation around the practice team.[7] The brochure contained very little about doctors, but aimed to encourage the use of all members of the primary health-care team. Indeed, in a research survey of the patients who were given a practice brochure, in order to measure its worth, only 12 per cent had heard of a 'primary health-care team'. This despite the fact that they had been coming to our practice and seeing our team grow over many years. Furthermore, the survey discovered that 55 per cent of the established patients of the practice discovered something in the brochure that they had not realized was available. For example, 26 per cent did not know that a marriage counsellor worked at the practice premises; in fact she had been there for many years.[8] The brochure was given to 262 new and established patients. The overall reaction was that they liked it, thought it helpful, and thought it improved their knowledge of team care. To 30 per cent of both new and established patients, the main message of the brochure was 'don't bother the doctor unnecessarily', and to 30 per cent of new patients it was 'who to approach for information and service'. So the message of using the whole team and sparing the doctor certainly came across.

Two earlier chapters in this book have described for the benefit of doctor-readers how the team can work efficiently and what the potential of each member is (Chapters 1 and 2). The practice brochure does exactly that for patients. Hence there are sections about the various workers and how they can be used most effectively and efficiently. For example, the description of the receptionists in the brochure informs patients that the receptionists have been trained and that many of them are very experienced. To quote the brochure:

they have a lot of information at their fingertips and could probably answer many of your queries. Anything you tell them will be treated in absolute confidence. If you are unsure whether to consult your doctor, nurse or health visitor, etc., the receptionists will be able to advise you. If you are in doubt about anything, ask the receptionist. If she does not know the answer she will ask someone who does.

If patients follow this advice, all those somewhat useless administrative queries such as patients making appointments to have their passports signed or to have some administrative form completed, can be avoided.

Good, well-informed, helpful receptionists can be a major means of increasing the efficiency of the practice and decreasing inappropriate doctor consultations, and also inappropriate consultations with other clinical members of the team. We sometimes wonder if each doctor—and hence each personal list—should have his own receptionist. This would seem a logical extension of personal care, and as receptionist and patients using her services got to know each other better, trust would grow and efficiency increase. Experiments are needed.

The nurses

As I have intimated many times in this book, the nurses are fundamental and central to the working of the team. Hence it is not surprising that our practice brochure has several pages devoted to their activities. The general description of the nurses is as follows:

The nurses

There are both district nurses and practice nurses working at the Medical Centre and all of them are prepared to advise you if they feel your problem is within their training and competence. Please feel free to seek their advice any time—there is one on duty at the surgery almost throughout the entire working day and you can also make appointments to see a nurse.

   The nurses don't mind an occasional telephone call, so if you feel you want some really quick advice ring up and ask for nurse and she will probably be able to help you.

District nurses   The district nurses are particularly concerned with the continuing care of the older people in the practice. If you know of some old person who appears to you to be in need and has not seen anyone in the team for quite a while, please contact one of the nurses and she will deal with this.

   For any conditions involving dressings, injections, stitches (possibly after having been to hospital), make an appointment with the district nurse.

   The district nurses run clinics each morning for blood tests (so that the samples can be despatched for analysis at the Path Lab the same afternoon), and Monday to Thursday afternoon for other nursing procedures.

Practice nurses   The practice nurses run a series of clinics in the surgery. These clinics are busy, so if you can't keep an appointment please inform us as soon as possible so that it may be offered to someone else.

   After this general description of the nurses there then follow descriptions of the practice nurses' primary and secondary preventative-care clinics:

Well woman clinic   Well Woman Checks: Monday and Thursday afternoons and Friday mornings.

Cervical Smears only: Tuesday and Wednesday mornings.

We believe that every woman in the practice between the ages of 18 and 65 should have a cervical smear carried out about every three years. The practice nurse runs a clinic for this and if you feel you are due for a smear please ask to see her. At the same time you can discuss any anxieties you have about your health. The nurse will also teach you how to carry out a self-examination of your breasts and will do routine checks on blood pressure, urine and blood if this seems appropriate. The clinic is well worthwhile—do use it.

Well man clinic   Friday afternoons

Since we believe in equality of the sexes we have now established a Well Man Clinic! The practice nurse runs this for all men aged between 30 and 69, who are not attending the doctor regularly for a chronic illness. At the clinic the nurse will make enquiries about your general health, your occupation, your family history and your smoking, drinking and exercise habits. She will measure your height, weight and blood pressure and check your urine (bring an 'after meals' specimen along please). After that she will be able to tell you whether you are really well and if you are not, what you should be doing about it. Obviously if she picks up any medical problems she will send you to see your doctor. You should have a Well Man Check every five years.

Diabetic clinic   Thursday mornings

By and large we try to look after the diabetics in our practice ourselves and save a lot of out-patient time not to mention a lot of patient time going there.

We have a diabetic clinic run by one of our nurses and there is a dietitian available at the same time. If at these routine sessions problems are detected then referral to the doctor is organized.

You will be given a diabetic booklet in which your diabetic notes will be kept so that you have a continuous record of how you are.

So if you are a diabetic, you should be coming to our diabetic clinic.

Vascular clinic   Thursday mornings

High blood pressure, narrowing and hardening of the arteries, angina, heart attacks, strokes—are all commonplace these days and very much inter-related. Our practice nurses are specially trained to carry out many of the tests and investigations and much of the routine care of people with these sorts of conditions, so don't be surprised if you find yourself having regular blood pressure checks, urine and blood tests by the practice nurse, if you come into one of these categories.

But remember, preventative care in vascular disease has a great deal to offer. If you attend the Well Woman or Well Man Clinic regularly, and take the advice the nurses give you, then you'll probably never get to the Vascular Clinic.

There is no doubt that patients with appropriate conditions, on reading the above, would be able to attend their doctor less.

Family planning, menopause, and HRT clinic, are also highlighted in the practice brochure, as follows:

Family planning   Clinics are run by the Family Planning Sister and are held Tuesday afternoons until 6 p.m. and Wednesday mornings until 12 noon. It is necessary to make appointments for these sessions.

All methods of contraception are available including the pill, the coil, the cap and injectable methods. Regular six-monthly or yearly check-ups are recommended according to the method used. Please make sure that once a year you complete a family planning form.

Pre-conception counselling   If you are thinking of having a baby there are various matters to be checked over before you conceive. Just make an appointment for a pre-conception counselling session with the family planning nurse.

Menopause and HRT Clinic   Symptoms of the menopause and what to do about them are common problems. One of our nurses has studied this area particularly, and will be glad to talk to you and advise. Patients using HRT (hormone replacement therapy) should have a check with the nurse about once a year.

Health visitors   Discussion with health visitors can include a wide variety of topics; infant feeding, speech development, immunisation, two year tantrums, minor illnesses (for example colds, sticky eyes, napkin rashes) etc., etc.

The health visitors can also provide information about local facilities such as mothers' groups, playgroups and day nurseries.

The system of hearing and developmental tests is organized and carried out by a health visitor on all children under 5.

The best time to contact your health visitor is between 9.00 and 10.00 a.m., and between 4.00 and 4.30 p.m. (telephone 360111). She will be pleased to discuss any health concerns you might have and provide information on specific health needs.

The dietitian   Once a week a hospital-based dietitian visits the practice and runs a dietetic clinic. If you are on a special diet for a medical condition please see her from time to time. If you are merely overweight or underweight it may be worthwhile consulting her to see what you should be doing about it but, at the end of the day, the answer to the problem lies very much in your own hands. Don't forget that extra exercise is just as important as dieting when you are trying to lose weight.

Please let us know if you can't attend an appointment with the dietitian; we want to make the best use of her limited and valuable time in the medical centre.

And so the practice brochure goes on, describing the other team members—midwife, counsellor, social workers, community psychiatric nurses, and so on—giving a general description of their work and a detailed account of their availability.

It is not surprising, therefore, that when the statistical survey of the value of the practice brochure was carried out, the 262 new and established patients who had read a copy of the brochure, when asked how they would respond to certain hypothetical health problems and clinical situations, made significantly greater use of the non-doctor members of the team than the matched sample who had not read it. Furthermore, inappropriate use of members of the team was not engendered. Various 'catch' questions had been inserted into the questionnaire in an attempt to elicit this.

The practice brochure certainly seemed to encourage a more appropriate use of services, hence saving a considerable amount of doctors' time not to mention decreasing a certain amount of doctors' irritation. The second-commonest theme that patients identified in the brochure was 'don't bother the doctor unnecessarily', while 42 per cent of established patients and 45 per cent of new patients thought that the brochure's most important message was to 'consult other members of the team (rather than the doctor)'. Thus, doctors' work-load falls yet the comprehensiveness and quality of the care improves.

Perhaps more mention should be made in the brochure of the new-style practice managers now present in the larger groups.[9,10] The current entry states:

Practice manager: responsible for the overall provision of clinics, staff, building maintenance and supplies, as well as dealing with the financial and legal side of the practice.

Perhaps it should go on to say something about the practice manager being available to listen to any complaints from patients; this gives patients the opportunity to let off steam and the manager the opportunity to defuse the situation. In our own practice the practice manager has, on one or two occasions in the last few years, probably prevented patients taking medico-legal action.

Central to everything is the team. So early in the brochure there occurs this description:

The primary health care team The team is made up of some forty people and includes doctors, different sorts of nurses, health visitors, social workers, a counsellor and MacMillan nurses, as well as administrative staff such as the practice manager, the computer/research secretary, the receptionists and, of course YOU!

Your own personal team will comprise those people relevant to your particular problem at any given time and its members will change according to your needs.

The doctors, nurses and other members of the team meet every morning to discuss patients' clinical problems. Each member of the team is well aware of the expertise of his fellow workers and from time to time seeks another opinion or can ask for their advice.

Particularly when the work-load is heavy the team shares out the work in order to get it carried out in the most effective manner.

But to correct the impression that the brochure is merely an attempt to turn off all patients from their doctors, here is the description which immediately follows:

Your 'own personal' doctor   There will be one doctor in the group that you and your family will look upon as your 'own' personal doctor. You will get to know each other well and it will usually be advantageous to wait until he or she is available. Occasionally, your doctor will be away on a course or on holiday. If your problem is urgent and you can't wait, the receptionist will arrange for you to see one of the other doctors who will look after you until your own doctor is back again.

Clearly the brochure must avoid giving the impression that the doctor never wants to see his patients, or that patients should see him again and again for inappropriate problems that can be better dealt with by other team members.

Information about activities

Also in the practice brochure are descriptions of the various activities in which patients can become involved. There is particular mention of the patients' group which meets once a month during the non-summer months and has discussions on various health matters, not necessarily merely relating to the practice.[11,12] There is also information about the practice newsletters which appear from time to time, and patients are exhorted to read these.

Details of the practice library, and who to see about borrowing and how to borrow books is also contained in the brochure.[13,14]

'Instructions' in the practice brochure

Because of the prevalence of minor illness and the opportunity, by reducing it, to reduce the number of consultations per patient, the practice brochure contains half a page of text near the beginning on this subject:

Minor illness   Many people treat their own minor illness—coughs, colds, diarrhoea, aches and pains, etc.—by going to the chemist for medicines. We think this is correct and by doing this you will leave the practice team free to cope with more serious problems. Chemists know a lot about minor remedies so consult the chemist first but if your symptoms persist then contact your own doctor. Don't forget that if something is troubling you but you are unsure whether to bother the doctor or not, make an appointment with the nurse who may well solve the problem . . .

. . . Everyone worries about 'leaving things too late'. We virtually never see this. But we do see a lot of people who come too early, either before we can make a diagnosis or before they have given the illness a chance to get better on its own.

Do note that this second paragraph under the heading of minor illness explodes one of the common myths of medical-school training—that early diagnosis is all-important. Patently it has advantages for the more significant pathological illnesses, such as breast-lumps, sudden paralyses, chest pain, or acute earache, but it does not refer to the common-or-garden, obvious respiratory infections which are constantly endemic, and at times epidemic, in the community. Unfortunately the medical-school myth has seeped into the conventional wisdom of society, and premature presentation of these self-limiting illnesses is commonplace.

You will note also the encouragement to use the chemists as experts and, if not the chemists, then perhaps a nurse. Later in the brochure there is a reference to non-prescribing which can ultimately be so cost- and time-effective (see Chapter 5):

Prescriptions and prescribing   Many illnesses get better on their own. All you often need is some reassurance that what you have got is indeed truly minor—and some general advice about your routine until it gets better. Pills and medicine are often completely unnecessary. Be prepared to leave the surgery without a prescription. Don't forget to use the chemist as we suggest in the section on 'Minor Illness'.

The practice brochure also contains 'dos and don'ts', and advice about how to use the services effectively (for example, not to call an ambulance in an acute illness and only to go directly to Accident and Emergency departments for trauma or in cases of poisoning). Instructions on how to get repeat prescriptions are spelled out clearly:

Repeat prescriptions   If you are taking regular medication you can obtain repeat prescribing through the receptionists. You will be given a computer slip listing your medication which you should use when requesting repeats. Please allow at least 24 hours for the prescription to be made out—longer if you need any alteration to your medication or it is time for it to be reviewed. Alternatively send a stamped addressed envelope and the prescription will be sent by post.

We do not take telephone orders for repeat prescriptions. Mistakes do occur that way. For people living a long way from the surgery the postal system is probably the best.

Please don't ask your doctor to write out your repeat prescription since the great majority of these are on the surgery computer—and the computer has more time than your doctor and is certainly more accurate!

Using the surgery

The practice brochure too gives an opportunity to instruct patients about surgery times, including mentioning that the Saturday morning surgery is for emergencies only. Opportunities for receiving advice in the evenings and at night from the duty doctor can be described. Some practices produce a separate card for this purpose which probably includes the practice telephone numbers, but we have amalgamated all these things into the one practice brochure. Advice on when to telephone, and for what is given—requests for visits early in the morning, appointments later in the morning, and general information (blood-test results, and so on) preferably in the afternoon. Examples of what constitutes an urgent appointment can be described (acute earache, chest pain, and so on).

Giving appropriate information about home visits is important. Patients tend to overrate this system, and while at times it is valuable it must not be overdone. In our practice brochure home visits merit half a page:

Home visits   These take a long time so do try to get to the surgery if you can. If you can't manage it under your own steam there is usually somebody around (a friend, a neighbour, a relative) who can give you a lift down in a car. Do remember, if you happen to be a car driver, that one of the good turns you can do an old person is to offer to transport them to the doctors when they are feeling ill or for their routine consultation.

If you really need a home visit, please put the call in before 10 a.m. on the day you want the visit and give as much detail of the problem as possible to the receptionist, since some visits are carried out by the nursing staff if this seems appropriate.

However, if an emergency arises during the day the receptionists will ensure that you are put in touch with the duty doctor.

Note that in this paragraph there is special mention of the elderly since, as intimated earlier, it is they who receive the largest number of home visits in any practice (see Chapter 3).[15]

The benefits of the telephone are also spelled out in the practice brochure:

Telephone advice   Sometimes you may feel that all you need is a quick word with someone on the telephone. Start by asking the receptionist; if she cannot help then she will put you through to the appropriate person—nurse, health visitor, midwife, doctor, etc.

A good time to ring is before 10 a.m. If the person you need is consulting, the receptionist will take details and we will ring back at a specific time.

You can often save yourself and your doctor a lot of time and effort by using the telephone in place of a visit or appointment, and we don't mind at all.

Thus, many of the principles of efficient care spelled out earlier in this book are relayed to the patients in the practice brochure. In the rapidly moving practice which is always trying to expand its services and improve the care, the practice brochure will go out of date. For example, in our own an attempt was made to describe a 'new-patient clinic' in the first and second editions. Unfortunately the clinic did not prove too successful, and in the third edition it was omitted. However, with the mandatory regulation in the 'new contract' that all patients over the age of 5 should be offered an introductory interview with the practice on registration, a new-patient clinic has now been re-established. Obviously the forthcoming fourth edition of the brochure will include this again. But the authors of the brochure can be happy that it does become out of date, as evidence that the practice is a constant hive of activity.

ANNUAL REPORT

It is now obligatory for general practitioners to produce an annual report, and the government's intention under the rules of the 'new contract' was that they would be made available to FHSAs. However, there seems little reason why these reports should not also be made available to patients in the practice, although much of the information will be fairly meaningless to them (probably as meaningless as it will be to the FHSAs!) Details of what is required can be obtained from the regulations themselves, but basically the reports indicate the number of staff other than doctors assisting the doctor in his practice, with their principal duties, hours of work, qualifications, and training. Implicit here is the suggestion that the members of the staff *are* trained, and in the efficient practice this of course is vital. There then has to follow an account of the practice premises, plus an account of all the referrals to in-patients and out-patients by specialty. Patients reading this with no frame of reference will be somewhat confused, and even more so when they look at the numbers of referrals to X-ray, pathology, and so on. The doctors also have to provide an account of their other commitments as medical practitioners, and the amount of time they spend on them. They also have to describe 'the nature of any arrangements whereby the doctor, or his staff, receive patients' comments on his provision of general medical services'. Finally, an account has to be given of the drugs and appliances that the doctors prescribe, and whether they use their own separate formulary. Even in this somewhat sterile document, aspects of efficiency rear their not-too-ugly heads.

PRACTICE NEWSLETTERS

The practice newsletter can come out as frequently as those involved have the time and energy to produce it. Usually, it falls to the practice manager to organize its contents, and in our own practice it appears approximately quarterly. Drug firms seem to be prepared to pay for the printing of the newsletters—certainly in our case. One purpose of the newsletter is to update or amend the brochure and reinforce efforts to increase the efficient use of the practice. In addition, it contains practice 'news'. In a recent newsletter of ours the following were the main items:

(1) notification of one doctor having left and another taking his place; the names of the trainees and for whom they were working; one or two staff changes;

(2) changes in the telephone number, in surgery times, and an announcement of closing of the surgery for staff training on Thursday lunchtimes for two hours;

(3) the role of the receptionist was described—by a receptionist;

(4) the protocol for well-person clinics was reiterated, the text being taken from the practice brochure (not everyone reads it, and repetition in any case is probably helpful);

(5) what was happening at the Patients' Group and the Asthma Group;

(6) a drug-and-alcohol abuse clinic being set up; also a tranquillizer-withdrawal group.

SELF-HELP GROUPS

Just as, in a school, pupils learn more from each other than they do from their teachers, so patients can learn more from each other than they can from their doctors. For example, at smoking groups patients can support, encourage, and teach each other how to stop smoking, and at a weight-watchers people help each other to lose weight. The most successful example of a self-help group in my own practice was the asthma group. This was initiated by popular request, from the patients' group. All young asthmatics and the parents of asthmatic children were written to. Patients' names were obtained from the practice disease index, and supplemented (the practice index not as yet being totally reliable) by the names of people receiving repeat prescriptions for asthma medication. Notices were displayed in the waiting areas in the surgery, and the asthma group was mentioned in successive newsletters. The practice brochure also contains some information about it. The response was extremely good and the number of asthmatics, or parents of asthmatics, attending varied between ten and fifteen. The group met monthly for about three years, but ultimately ceased since it had achieved its aims for that particular group of people. There is no doubt that the knowledge of asthma amongst the sufferers in the practice improved considerably, and doctors in their consulting-rooms soon became aware of this. To say that several of us felt a little threatened at times by the patients' knowledge is an understatement. Patients' expectation of their health rose, and they could no longer be fobbed off with a woolly account of, for example, the use of the various types of inhaler, spacer, turbohaler, nebuhaler, nebuliser, and so on. By improved knowledge of their disease, the patients then educated the doctor!

Currently, having had their care of asthma improved, the doctors are considering whether to form 'eczema groups' and 'psoriasis groups'. One possibility resulting from these groups is the establishment of special clinics, ultimately to be run by nurses, for the ongoing care of these conditions.

INVOLVING PATIENTS FROM THE PATIENT'S POINT OF VIEW

It seems from my experience, and even as a matter of principle, that patients prefer a democratic system in which they feel involved. It is no longer 'them' (health-care workers) and 'us' (the patients). The feeling to be engendered is of doctor and patient working together against ill health and disease. Patients like information. Many of them do read newsletters, brochures, and hand-outs about their illnesses, and find them of interest. In the future they will read the annual report! It will raise their expectations, and in the United Kingdom patients' expectations have always been far too low. Our patients, both new and old, liked the practice brochure, as evidenced statistically from the associated survey. It provides them with a guide to easy and efficient care which they can understand and with which they can comply. Because consulting-room memories are short, clinical hand-outs are popular. The self-help groups have been a great success, especially the asthma one. New patients who come into the practice mostly welcome the interest taken in them by having to complete an appropriate form; most of them are happy to have a nurse interview. Since many newly registering patients simultaneously wish to consult their new doctor, he too can follow the 'new-patient' protocol. This also seems to go down well.

REFERENCES

1. Marsh, G. N. (1972). Controversial view: 'back to single-handed.' *RCGP North-east Faculty Newsletter*.
2. Gray, D. J. Pereira (1979). The key to personal care. *Journal of the Royal College of General Practitioners*, **29**, 666–78.
3. British Medical Association (1986). *General practitioner services: GMSC's guidelines on practice booklets*. London.
4. Mead, M. (1990). How to produce a practice leaflet. *Update*, **40**, 137–40.

5. Neville, R. G. and Mason, C. (1987). The evaluation of a general practice patient information leaflet: a pilot study. *Health Bulletin*, **45**, 185–9.
6. Monopolies and Mergers Commission (1989). *Services of medical practitioners: a report on the supply of the services of registered medical practitioners in relation to restrictions on advertising*. HMSO, London.
7. Marsh, G. N. (1980). The practice brochure: a patient's guide to team care. *British Medical Journal*, **281**, 730–2.
8. Marsh, G. N. and Barr, J. (1975). Marriage guidance counselling in a group practice. *Journal of the Royal College of General Practitioners*, **25**, 73–5.
9. Huntington, J., Irvine, S., and Marinker, M. (1987). *Management in practice*. Video and course book. RCGP/MSD Foundation, London.
10. Drury, M. (ed.) (1990). *The new practice manager*. Radcliffe, Oxford.
11. Pritchard, P. (ed.) (1981). *Patient participation in general practice*. Occasional Paper 17. RCGP, London.
12. Richardson, A. and Bray, C. (1987). *Promoting health through participation: experience of groups for patient participation in general practice*. Policy Studies Institute, London.
13. Leverton, T. (1988). Practical steps to starting a patients' library. *Practitioner*, **232**, 1393–6.
14. Varnavides, C. K., Zermansky, A. G. and Pace, C. (1984). Health library for patients in general practice. *British Medical Journal*, **288**, 535–7.
15. Whewell, J., Marsh, G. N., and McNay, R. A. (1983). Changing patterns of home visiting in the north of England. *British Medical Journal*, **286**, 1259–61.

15. Having a trainee

INTRODUCTION

Although this chapter is not specifically designed to raise the hackles of those involved in the education of future general practitioners, it almost certainly will. It is written against the background of my own practice in which there are two trainers, one associate regional adviser, and, not infrequently, two trainee GPs. This has been the case for the last two years; prior to that there had been two trainers (one 'unemployed' for alternate six months) for approximately twenty years. The opinions which follow have also been substantiated by discussions with many trainers and trainees across the years.

There is no doubt that 'training is for education and not for changing work-load—at least that is the theory': so wrote an eminent professor of general practice when reviewing the proposed content of this book. Whether trainees do increase or decrease the work-load of their trainers is very debatable, but the overall conclusion from this chapter is that they decrease it.[1-4]

TYPE OF TRAINEE

The great majority of trainees know very little when they enter general practice for the first time. Their clinical experience is extremely limited, their attitudes are usually narrow, and they find difficulty in relating to patients. There are, of course, enormous differences between the junior trainee who is just starting and the senior trainee who has already done six months in general practice. In some training programmes the trainee does one continuous twelve-month session, so presumably he gradually changes into a more mature doctor by the end of his time in practice. And there are both good and bad medical graduates entering general practice. Patently all these differences will affect whether their contribution to practice work-load is positive or negative. But in this chapter I shall try to consider the average trainee who is keen to learn and gain experience, and who is hoping ultimately to get a good reference from his trainer and his course organizer.

THE TRAINEE'S DRAIN ON THE TRAINER

As well as providing an efficient consulting-room (see Chapter 11), the facilities, and the supporting staff (see Chapters 1 and 2), the trainer has to provide moment-to-moment support for problems which the trainee meets and cannot deal with. In the early consulting sessions of the first few weeks of the junior trainee's experience, he will bring the trainer records of the patients he has seen. These are discussed in detail. Initially the trainer will need to take the trainee on home visits, and particularly 'chronic' visits, with the ultimate aim of handing over three or four 'chronic' visits to the trainee for his time in the practice. My recent trainee has just taken over the continuing care of an elderly, bedroom-bound, chronic bronchitic and asthmatic whose medicated survival has improved since the invention of the nebuliser, as well as a house-bound, alcoholic, arachnophobe whose life has been ruined by spiders, and an osteo-arthritic couple, one with stasis ulcers to the leg, the other with chronic peptic ulceration and Paget's disease. The trainer will accompany the trainee on night-calls for the first three or four months in the practice. Thereafter he is available when the trainee does night-calls alone. In my practice each trainer spends two hours per week in face-to-face tutorials with the trainee or trainees.[5,6] Each trainee also has a thirty-minute consulting session in front of a two-way mirror with his trainer observing; this is followed by a discussion as to what has transpired.[7] The trainer, trainee, and other partners in the practice take part in weekly analyses of video-recorded consultations by any of them.[8,9] Each trainee answers a 450-question multiple-choice paper twice during a six-month appointment. He is also set one essay question every six weeks. Multiple-choice questions and essays are marked by the trainer.

The above commitments make a considerable volume of work for the trainer: it would not seem unreasonable for him to expect some reduction of work-load in return.

HOW TRAINEES EASE THE WORK-LOAD

Trainees need to see patients and so they have regular surgeries, although they are often not fully booked. Thus they can look after a few patients at their own speed: simultaneously the trainer's work-load falls. As their experience increases they do unaccompanied acute home visits on their trainer's patients, and also do continuing 'chronic' visits on the patients he allocates to them. Again the trainer's work-load falls. They are also available to respond to the 'semi-urgent' request for a home visit, often to the far edge of the practice, in the middle of a surgery session. Similarly, they reduce the trainer's tiring home visits late in the day and, as they become more experienced, also in the evening and night. Senior trainees can take their place on the rota, so long as a partner is available to cover them; thus they reduce not only the trainer's work but also that of the whole practice.

THE NET RESULT OF ALL THIS

Overall, the trainer does fewer attendances and visits. The 'leg-weariness', particularly of the older trainer, is reduced by an energetic young trainee. Some senior trainees can take over their trainer's entire practice for limited periods—say a fortnight at a time—and the trainer remains in the background as a resource person. Hence the trainee can try his hand at taking on almost total responsibility.

I think I must conclude, having pondered all this, that a trainer will be more able to cope efficiently for 3000 patients on his list with the help of an average trainee (junior or senior) than he would without one. And simultaneously he would be able to train his trainee adequately.

HAVING A TRAINEE FROM THE PATIENT'S POINT OF VIEW

Some patients welcome trainees, particularly mothers of young children who feel that they are 'never away' from the surgery with the recurring minor illnesses of their children. To be able to see someone other than their own doctor comes almost as a relief. Trainees work at a slower pace and can give patients plenty of time to talk; this is welcome. Patients also enjoy being able to recap on chronic problems which they are reluctant to repeat to their own doctor, who has heard them so many times before. They also approach trainees as young doctors with the 'latest knowledge' from teaching centres, who may possibly have new or different ideas. Some perceptive patients realize that trainees bring an academic stimulus into a practice, and also that training practices have to subscribe to certain standards. Such patients will see the practice as being 'better' than practices that have not been accredited for training.

REFERENCES

1. Pearson, C. R. and Goss, B. M. (1989). Comparison of the work-load of a trainer and trainee. *Journal of the Royal College of General Practitioners*, **39**, 320–3.

2. Crawley, H. S. and Levin, J. B. (1990). Training for general practice: a national survey. *British Medical Journal*, **300**, 911–15.
3. Fleming, D. M. (1986). A comparison of the practice activities of trainees and principals. *Journal of the Royal College of General Practitioners*, **36**, 212–16.
4. Carney, T. A. (1987). Trainee work-load—are we winning the battle? *Horizons*, **1**, 481–4.
5. Ronalds, C., Douglas, A., Gray, D. J. P., and Selby, P. (1981). *Fourth National Trainee conference. Report, Recommendations and Questionnaire. Exeter 1980.* Occasional Paper 18. RCGP, London.
6. Gray, D. J. P. (1982). *Training for general practice*. MacDonald and Evans, Plymouth.
7. Elliott, B., Marsh, G. N., Strachan, D., and Cooke, J. (1979). Patients' reactions to a two-way mirror in general practice. *Medical Education*, **13**, 439–42.
8. Roberts, G. D. (1985). Using videotapes to teach the consultation. *Trainee*, **5** (**2**), 67–9.
9. Pringle, M., Robins, S., and Brown, G. (1984). Assessing the consultation: methods of observing trainess in general practice. *British Medical Journal*, **288**, 1659–60.

16. From greater efficiency to larger lists

Each chapter in this book has spelled out the resultant benefits of being efficient in various aspects of practice work. But although efficiency can be regarded as a quality, it is not an end in itself. So what are the results of all this efficiency—indeed why bother? Is it worth it? Of paramount importance is that efficiency provides the doctor with more time—time for study, teaching, audit, research, and for thinking about, and ultimately implementing the expansion of services—all self-evident benefits. But it also provides him with more time for more patients, should he feel so inclined. So, in this final chapter, let me consider list-size.

During the 1970s and 1980s, the average number of patients on doctors' lists fell from approximately 3000 per doctor to 2000.[1] And yet during this period the numbers of team colleagues increased; in general terms 'productivity' fell, as measured by the number of patients looked after per health-care worker. It would seem that the government, probably rightly, felt that list-sizes had fallen as far as they should, and that there should now be some incentive to increase the number of patients cared for: hence the greater emphasis in the 'new contract' on payment for numbers of patients.[2] There has been a continuing and inconclusive debate across the years as to whether doctors with smaller lists give better care.[3-5] The arguments have been confused, particularly because there are few parameters of quality of care. There seems to be some evidence that doctors with smaller lists attend more assiduously and more effectively to preventative care,[6] but this book would question this 'quality', preventative care being largely a nursing task (see Chapter 7).

Has a large list any virtues in itself? I believe it has. Having had a personal list of around 3000 patients for most of my working life, and in my middle years allowing this to rise to 4200 patients (helped by a trainee, and hence without undue stress and strain), and now with the enthusiasm and energy to continue practising into my sixties, I feel perhaps appropriately experienced to substantiate my views.

Greater job satisfaction can flow from a larger rather than a smaller list. To care for a larger number of people imbues one with a comfortable feeling of doing more for society. Put simplistically, if a doctor in a small town of 3000 people looks after every one of them, his standing in the community is much greater than if he shares that population with two or three colleagues. He has an overall greater sphere of influence. He can be proud of his greater productivity and the greater return on the several thousands of pounds invested in him during his training. He can also feel a greater return on all the hours of intensive hard work which ultimately got him into his practice. It is also a greater return on all his teachers' work. From a negotiating point of view, if each doctor has a large list of patients, it gives them greater power than if they had only a small number of people dependent on them. So in terms of self-esteem, assuming that the quality of care is satisfactory, large lists can be good for doctors.

The more patients, the more clinical material: this is somewhat self-evident, but consider an illness whose prevalence in the community is, say, 1 per cent—for example, diabetes. In a list of 2000 patients there would be twenty diabetics; in a list of 3000 there would be thirty. Expertise from experience of these people would increase half as much again with the larger list. But illnesses vary in their degree and type, so the larger number of patients would give larger numbers of each type of diabetic.

One of the reasons given for dwindling intra-partum care by general practitioners is that the number of normal deliveries in a list of 2000 patients of average age-distribution is only approximately ten to fifteen per year[7]—only just enough to maintain skills. If the number rose to 3000, then there would be half as many births again. And so this argument can prevail across the whole spectrum of health care. Even the diagnosis of rare diseases (for example, acute appendicitis or perforated peptic ulcer) becomes marginally easier if they occur once or twice per year rather than every two or three years. So, more clinical material—enjoyable in itself—means that experience of less-common illnesses grows and that GPs can maintain their expertise.

Relatively common illnesses like asthma, hypertension, diabetes, depression, angina, irritable bowel syndrome, and peptic ulcer become the commonplace 'stuff' of clinically rewarding general practice, and more easily so with the larger list. Even the special practical skills necessary for intra-natal care, minor ops sessions, insertion of intra-uterine devices, and fitting of diaphragms can all be kept refreshed with a greater number of patients. Paradoxically, the more clinical problems one has of a particular condition the fewer one needs to send to hospital, since experience, confidence, and expertise will all rise simultaneously. Even for less-common problems, those in group practices can develop some 'specialoid' system whereby one partner takes a specific interest in a particular area such as minor ops or Ventouse deliveries. This work would be much better executed by a partner than it would be at the local hospital, where it would mostly be done by junior staff in training.

Implicit in all this, of course, is that the number of consultations per patients per year must fall. A large number of the relatively minor and unimportant consultations will cease as a result of many of the ideas in this book. Does this matter? Will doctors not know their patients as well? As I mentioned in the Introduction, it was anxiety about this that made me undertake a patient-satisfaction survey in the mid-1970s.[8,9] I was only seeing patients on average 2.3 times per year, compared with an overall national figure of 3.5 to 4.5 times.[10] Were patients missing me? Did they feel neglected? Was I becoming unpopular? Could they only see me when I was on television!

To cut a long story short, and summarize a very comprehensive and detailed survey, patient satisfaction was extremely high. Most important of all was that, patients were not only highly satisfied with their doctor but were simultaneously highly satisfied with the care by other team members.[9] Bear in mind that from a numerical point of view, a patient with a serious illness, for example a newly diagnosed depression or thyroid deficiency, will be seen frequently by his general practitioner anyway; to some extent the averages are meaningless. It is well known that a very small percentage of patients produce a large proportion of the consultations. In my own practice 13 per cent of patients had 50 per cent of the consultations in one year.[10] So, although the overall figures of 2.3 consultations versus 3.5 to 4.5 seem wildly different, it is probable that patients with serious illness will be seen only a little less frequently, and will not notice this. When a child in a family is seen, because it attends with a member of its family this equates virtually with two consultations, although only one clinical problem is dealt with. Similarly, care of elderly dependent relatives flows over into care of the carers and others in the household. The average consultation-rate per family will be very much higher than 2.3 per family per year. And as we have seen, less-frequent consultations can become longer and more meaningful—truly clinically satisfying.

Larger numbers of patients necessitate a multi-disciplinary team, and as this team materializes the doctor's satisfaction in sharing and discussing problems with a varied group of co-workers becomes considerable. The team members illuminate aspects of the problem which may not have been apparent to him, and the patients receive broader and more comprehensive care. All this makes the doctor more satisfied with the work he is doing.

Efficiency produces more time for teaching, as well as time in which to prepare that teaching—and as part of the working day, not in the weary hours of the evening. But perhaps more important is the fact that with more patients there is more clinical material on which to teach. Varied diabetic clinics and vascular clinics containing all types of hypertension and ischaemic heart disease (not to mention the occasional rarity of an aortic aneurysm or a valvular heart disease) all provide more material for a greater breadth of teaching. In large practices, with say 15 000 patients and five partners, even rarities like Addisons's disease, carcinoid tumour, or phaeocromocytoma will be found. One of the reasons for six months' internal medicine for GP trainees at senior house-officer level is for them to be exposed to a concentration of clinical problems not only on the ward but, perhaps more importantly, at the out-patient department. The continuing-care clinics of large-list practices will become the future 'out-patient departments', and the educational material available at them will be considerable. Not only will trainers teach trainees, but medical students too will be attached as part of their undergraduate curriculum. The carefully ordered physical examination of patients and the elicitation of physical signs, an important part of undergraduate learning, will be possible in the doctor's surgery. So, efficiency gives more time for teaching and more material on which to teach, and this gives greater satisfaction for the teaching GPs.

As I mentioned earlier, the major change in the method of remunerating general practitioners moving from the old contract to the new has been the greater emphasis on capitation payment.[2] More patients means greater income. But more patients also means more items of service—more family planning, antenatal, intranatal, postnatal, and immunization fees—and more remuneration from more health-promotion clinics for more people. There is no doubt that most general practitioners' incomes have already risen under the 'new contract', but the conventional wisdom seems to be that those in large-list, efficient practices have risen disproportionately more. Discerning readers will note, and sensitive readers will be pleased, that I have left the financial rewards for the efficient large list until the end. But to me, enhanced clinical care, better teaching opportunities, and more research possibilities—all the elements of great job satisfaction—dwarf the extra financial return. However, if the income does seem to be high then the large-list doctor, giving good, efficient care, need not feel in any way embarrassed by it.

But not every GP is a megalomaniac and workaholic! The great majority of them have homes, families, gardens, hobbies, and the like. In the efficient practice there will be more time for these too, and doctors will find themselves, on at least four of the working days in the week, leaving the surgery at the latest by 5.30 or 6 p.m., well satisfied with a rewarding day's work.

THE LARGE LIST FROM THE PATIENT'S POINT OF VIEW

Whether the doctor has a large or a small list is immaterial to the patient, so long as she can be seen as promptly as is appropriate and given an efficient and caring service. If the doctor seems to be happy in his work, clinically interested, and rewarded, and at the end of the day enjoys a good financial return, then all this will rebound to the patient's advantage. Contented, fulfilled, and rewarded doctors make patients happy too. QED.

REFERENCES

1. Department of Health (1990). Statistics for general medical practitioners in England and Wales: 1978 to 1988. *Statistical Bulletin*, **4**, 9, 15.
2. Department of Health and Welsh Office (1989). *General practice in the national health service: a new contract*. DOH, London.
3. Roland, M. (1987). Is there a case for smaller lists? *Journal of the Royal College of General Practitioners*, **37**, 481-2.
4. Knight, R. (1987). The importance of list size and consultation length as factors in general practice. *Journal of the Royal College of General Practitioners*, **37**, 19-22.
5. Butler, J. R. and Calnon, M. W. (1987). List size and use of time in general practice. *British Medical Journal*, **245**, 1383-6.
6. Fleming, D. M., Lawrence, M. S. T. A., and Cross, K. W. (1985). List size, screening methods and other characteristics of practices in relation to preventive care. *British Medical Journal* **291**, 869-72.
7. Marsh, G. N., Cashman, H. A., and Russell, I. T. (1985). General practitioner participation in intranatal care in the Northern Region in 1983. *British Medical Journal*, **290**, 971-3.
8. Kaim-Caudle, P. R. and Marsh, G. N. (1975). Patient satisfaction survey in general practice. *British Medical Journal*, **1**, 262-4.
9. Marsh, G. N. and Kaim-Caudle, P. (1976). *Team care in general practice*. Croom Helm, London.
10. Marsh, G. N. (1974). *Team work-load in general practice*. Unpublished MD thesis. University of Newcastle upon Tyne.

Index

160   *Index*